Praise for

BEYOND AYAHUASCA

"Beyond Ayahuasca *is a rite of passage to help the
modern world transcend the many imposed limitations
that are separating us from our truest nature.*"

— **Nick Polizzi,** founder of The Sacred Science

T0357159

BEYOND AYAHUASCA

Hay House Titles of Related Interest

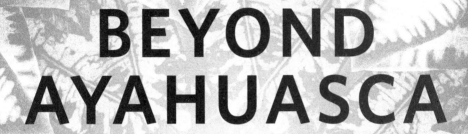

BEYOND AYAHUASCA

Unlocking the Evolutionary
Science of Indigenous
Amazonian Wisdom to Access
Your Highest Potential

ROMAN HANIS

HAY HOUSE LLC
Carlsbad, California • New York City
London • Sydney • New Delhi

Copyright © 2025 by Roman Hanis

Published in the United States by:
Hay House LLC: www.hayhouse.com®
P.O. Box 5100, Carlsbad, CA, 92018-5100

Cover design: Jordan Wannemacher • *Interior design:* Karim J. Garcia
Interior photos courtesy of the author.

Cataloging-in-Publication Data is on file at the Library of Congress

Tradepaper ISBN: 978-1-4019-7959-1
E-book ISBN: 978-1-4019-7960-7
Audiobook ISBN: 978-1-4019-7961-4

10 9 8 7 6 5 4 3 2 1
1st edition, May 2025

Printed in the United States of America

This product uses responsibly sourced papers, including recycled materials and materials from other controlled sources.

The authorized representative in the EU for product safety and compliance is Penguin Random House Ireland, Morrison Chambers, 32 Nassau Street, Dublin D02 YH68, Ireland. https://eu-contact.penguin.ie

CONTENTS

FOREWORD

Fifteen years ago, my team and I were in the early planning stages of a documentary on Amazonian Shamanism, *The Sacred Science*, scouring the earth for a main character, a compelling setting, and a gripping plot. After a few months of chasing down dead-end leads, I found myself sitting on a cold yoga studio floor out in Brighton Beach, Brooklyn. A handful of us had made the trek out to a predominantly Russian-speaking neighborhood, braving cold November drizzle to hear a traveling curandero speak.

The person before us exuded a world-weary wisdom that fell in stark contrast with the youth in his face, as if he was returning from some other dimension that we had not experienced. The look of a person who had seen some things they could never unsee.

What struck me that night about Roman's "Knowledge of the Amazon" talk was how meticulously he crafted each word, as if he was conjuring the spirit of the medicine itself, to give a quick taste to all who watched and listened. As he wove together Amazonian creation myth, ethnobotanical methodology, and a heaping dose of entheogenic safety precaution, we knew that he was preparing us for what was to come—if we chose to participate in the hush-hush Grandmother and Grandfather ceremonies he would be hosting that weekend.

Roman warned us that while our Western culture of convenience may feel safe and abundant, it is governed by a paralyzing aversion to change and the discomfort that accompanies it. In stark contrast lies the Amazonian way of healing, which beckons us into the unknown, recognizing our deepest fears as portals into our highest potential.

It has been more than a decade since that fateful evening and Roman has led many a wayward soul to the spirit path. As his friend and co-conspirator, it has been a gift to watch his own evolution—from a passionate and at times mischievous young master, to the life-humbled being of light who wrote this book.

By embodying his place and purpose in this carnation, Roman has shown the lucky among us what the word *shaman/healer* means. He is a living bridge, between the ecstatic and at-times-harrowing cosmic abyss of the unseen and the dense, business-as-usual modern world that most of us inhabit.

In the throes of my first grandmother ceremony that weekend of late 2009, Roman said something to me that I believe is the essence of this book.

We had taken the jungle sacrament a few hours earlier, and I found myself crawling at a snail's pace, across a darkened room that had somehow turned onto its side. I came to rest in a quaking heap before the healer, amidst a swirling kaleidoscope of color and sound. A glowing hand stretched out through the storm and touched my shoulder.

"Nick. Sometimes we must break down in order to break through."

***

After that first encounter with Roman, a half-formed understanding began to emerge in my mind:

At the heart of every culture is a language. A web of words and symbols that forms a mental corollary of each person, place, thing, or action that we can think of. Real or imagined. Taken together, each strand of words in this web forms an idea or belief inside our mind, which we involuntarily overlay onto the observable world outside. This interweaving creates a seamless understanding of the way things are.

The degree to which this web of word strands—language— affects our ability to see the raw externality around us is almost impossible to say. After all, saying requires language and language coats the lens of our perception from infancy to old age. We learn it in order to communicate our experience, but in doing so, we inhibit our direct knowing of the thing itself.

We are social creatures, and to socialize requires an adherence to the syntactical conventions of the culture we are born into. We learn all the communicable symbols and sounds for the external phenomena that matter to our culture—we label everything, including ourselves.

Somehow, the mastery of this system of labels begins to pass as knowledge of the very things we're labeling.

When asked who we are, we often respond with our name. Asked again, we'll respond with our profession. Asked a third time, we start getting uncomfortable.

The sages and mystics have always known that to truly *know* something is far different than reciting a cascade of labels that society deems worthy of describing it. Language is a blessing and a curse, and can be used for both. We've forgotten this in our modern age, haphazardly regurgitating ideas that have no basis in lived experience.

We lay alone at night, tormented in the dark by a raging sea of competing words and notions—many of which do not wish us well. The line separating these thoughts from our tangible reality has become so thin that the body responds to both in the exact same way, leaving us depleted from constant fight or flight and little to no rest and repair.

Perhaps this is why meditation (making the words stop) and prayer (intentionally speaking beneficial word strands) are the cornerstones of every world religion, including the earliest known spiritual belief system—shamanism. Aside from the physical tools in their medicine bag, the shaman holds one core operating principle—to be the ultimate truth. *In order to heal the mind and body, one must learn to see beyond the illusion of who they think they are and what they think this is.*

This is the only way to transcend our personal prison of self-imposed limitation and open to the infinite possibility that awaits us.

Among the many sacred rules of the road, Roman has shown me that the rational mind and ego must become a humble servant, aiding our soul's journey through this life. His book *Beyond Ayahuasca* is a rite of passage to help the modern world transcend the many imposed limitations that are separating us from our truest nature. Selfishly speaking, I can't wait for the second book in this series to come out!

Nick Polizzi,
founder of The Sacred Science

PREFACE TO THE TEXT

IQUITOS, Abril del 2012.

Carta S/N. RH.2012.

A LA OPINION PÚBLICA.

El presente documento confirma que recibimos de forma Oficial y Honorable a Roman Hanis como parte de nuestra Tribu y religión Yahua; en el que ha sido recocido por la Tribu Yahua, con el que entabla una amistad de mas de nueve años, brindando su apoyo para el bienestar de la gente Indígena.

Roman Hanis ha sido adoptado por la Tribu Yahua, siguiendo los rituales de iniciación de la Cultura y Religión Indígena Yahua; con la misión de representar la cultura y religión de la Tribu a nivel mundial; así mismo en la creencia de Nuestro Señor Jesucristo.

Roman Hanis esta aprobado como Curandero y Líder Religioso, para hacer Ritos Curativos Religiosos con Plantas Medicinales y Sagradas como el Ayahuasca, San Pedro, Chiri Sanango, Ajo Sacha, Chuchuhuasi, Uña de Gato, entre otros; con la finalidad de difundir y compartir los beneficios del conocimiento ancestral y las costumbres de la Tribu Yahua para mundo.

ATENTAMENTE.

ANCELMO CAHUACHI FACHIN
Huella digital de la mano
derecha

MARCIAL CAMPOS MANUYAMA
Testigo a Ruego
Marcial Campos Manuyama

CERTIFICO: que, la huella digital dedo indice mano derecha que antecede de don ANCELMO CAHUACHI FACHIN, identificado con DNI Nº 05309427, así como la firma de don MARCIAL CAMPOS MANUYAMA, identificado con DNI Nº 05242025, quien firma a ruego de don ANCELMO CAHUACHI FACHIN, son autenticas, doy fe.- Iquitos, 14 de Abril del 2012.- - - - - - - - - - - - - - - - - - -

JOSE M. SALAZAR BERNEDO
NOTARIO ABOGADO

JOSE M. SALAZAR BERNEDO
Notaria Pública
de Mayno
IQUITOS - PERU

Translated Document:

"Year of the National Integration and Recognition of Our Diversity"
IQUITOS, April, 2012
Presentation S/N. RH. 2012.
FOR PUBLIC KNOWLEDGE.

Current document confirms that we have adopted Roman Hanis in an Official and Honorable form to be part of our Tribe and religion Yahua; in which he was rewoven by the Yahua Tribe throughout a bonding friendship of over 9 years, during which he had been providing support for the well-being of the Indigenous people.

Roman Hanis has been adopted by the Yahua Tribe, following the initiation rituals of the Culture and the Indigenous Religion of Yahua; with the mission to represent the culture and religion of our Tribe on the global level; in accordance with the belief in Our Lord Jesus Christ (legally required statement).

Roman Hanis is approved as a Healer and a Religious Leader, to perform Religious Healing Rites with Medicinal and Sacred Plants such as Ayahuasca, San Pedro, Chiric Sanango, Ajo Sacha, Chuchuhuasi, Uña de Gato, among others; with the purpose of promoting and sharing the benefits of ancestral wisdom and the customs of the Yahua Tribe with the world.

Attentively,
Ancelmo Cahuachi Fachin
Official representative of the Yahua Tribe
Fingerprint of the right hand
Marcial Campos Manuyama
Witness to the testimony
Fingerprint and signature

Certified: that, the fingerprint of the right hand pertaining to don Anselmo Cahuachi Fachin, identified with DNI N 05309427, and also the signature of don Marcial Campos Manuyama, identified with DNI N 05242025, who signs to testify for the authenticity of don Ancelmo Cahuachi Fachin, with good faith. Iquitos, April 14, 2012
JOSE M. SALAZAR BERNEDO NOTARY – ATTORNEY
IQUITOS PERÚ PUBLIC NOTARY OF MAYNAS PROVINCE

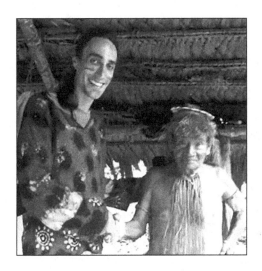

INTRODUCTION

The Evolutionary Science of Humanity

What does practical ancestral wisdom mean to you?

In the modern age of information overload, it's challenging to find a genuine wisdom lineage that can help us navigate life with a higher purpose. Yet, even finding a lineage is not enough, since that connection must be valued and honored, not used superficially to justify one's own unconscious, habitual behavior. We must consider how meaningful the lineage was to the ancestors of humanity who gave their lives to preserve it—and then, we must respect it accordingly.

Back in 2001, I was fortunate to meet a number of Amazonian elders who became my close lifelong friends and teachers. Although they shared with me the most profound instructions around the powerful Evolutionary Science behind their worldview and way of life, I do not view myself as being special. I simply ended up in the right place at the right time, with an illness that made me desperate enough to go through the arduous discipline of integrating the traditions of Amazonian plant medicine.

It has taken me more than 20 years to integrate the wisdom of South American ancestors, by applying it to my own healing journey and supporting many others on theirs. My life has been forever changed during my early encounters, and I hope that my story and what I learned will help you on your own journey.

Beyond Ayahuasca is a personal account of discovering a highly evolved ancestral civilization. I invite you, the reader, on an adventure to discover your innermost spark by immersing in the healing and self-realization journey of the traditions I have studied, which transcend many of the (currently commodified) Western ideas about South American spirituality—usually, ideas that are limited to the "Ayahuasca journey" but do not fully translate to the spectrum of spiritual wisdom that is such a vital part of this ancestral lineage.

A Living Tradition

The quest for healing and truth led me to question everything in my life at the most fundamental level. My conscious evolution began in 1998 with studies of diverse cognitive, holistic, and spiritual paths. These included transpersonal Jungian and Buddhist psychologies, Toltec teachings, psychedelic therapy and self-exploration, Tibetan Buddhism, and Traditional Chinese Medicine, among others.

As a culmination of an in-depth introduction into these disciplines, I was eventually led to the living wisdom traditions of the Amazon and Andes.

I first arrived in the Amazon rainforest in August 2001, guided by a series of synchronistic events. They included seemingly random books and people appearing in my life over a very short period of time, all pointing me to the Indigenous healing traditions of South America. I was undergoing both an existential and a health crisis at the time. In addition to the "incurable" illness I was facing, my first great love had married my best friend behind my back, and my successful attempt at a corporate career did nothing to win her back. I was disenchanted by "modern" life. There was nothing left for me to lose, and the perfect storm brewing in my life propelled me to abandon my conventional existence.

My gradual initiation into the mystery school of the Amazon rainforest took place under the guidance of wise elders, with whom I could relate as real human beings and friends. Moreover, perseverance on this path was largely due to my own incentive. Because of the severity of my health condition, I missed out on being a tourist collecting "exotic" experiences. Instead, I approached the South American precolonial traditions with the intention to heal an illness that was going to cut short my time on this Earth.

During my initial three years of formal healing apprenticeship, I lived in various Indigenous and *mestizo* (a term that denotes people with both Spanish and Indigenous lineages) communities. Fascinated by the culture, I explored many tributaries of the Amazon River, meeting various tribal elders and medicine men and women, some of whom became my lifelong teachers and friends. My studies intensified dramatically in 2004 when I was initiated as a *curandero* (healer) by the elder medicine man of the Yahua tribe. It's been an arduous yet fulfilling journey ever since.

The term *healer*, in its Indigenous connotation, is a life calling for someone who helps people discover their inherent healing potential by steadfastly cultivating their own. It is often true that those who undergo physical, emotional, and spiritual suffering and embark on a quest to heal it discover that their purpose is much larger. In finding healing, they unlock a more profound calling to aid others on similar journeys. You may find this to be true for yourself, as well.

In an earlier book on Amazonian Indigenous wisdom, *The Wizard of the Upper Amazon*, by Manuel Córdova-Rios and F. Bruce Lamb, a mysterious language of intuitive wisdom that includes telepathy is utilized by the Huni Kuin tribe, who live in Brazil and Peru. In his accounts, Córdova-Rios mentions the nearly impossible struggle he faced to meaningfully communicate what he had learned to his peers. Throughout my time living with the Indigenous and mestizo healers, I too have found myself greatly challenged in translating the ancestral wisdom into layman's terms. In this book, I attempt to share the multifaceted knowledge of the Amazonian ancestors in the most accurate and respectful way possible.

Where Cutting-Edge Science Meets Ancient Wisdom

The ancestors survived many calamities over countless generations by honoring the human spirit under the harshest of conditions. These lessons of adaptation and wisdom, so carefully gathered through the ages, are key for humanity to emerge from the current global crisis in which health and environmental disasters, war, famine, and other forms of catastrophic conflict are caused by the collective deterioration of human values.

Ironically, the blueprint of humanity's next evolutionary stage is hidden in the misinterpreted and overlooked. It's time for the sleeping giant of ancestral ingenuity to awaken.

Over the last few decades, fascinating evidence has been discovered about the precolonial history of the Amazon rainforest. Numerous recent findings have verified that the Amazon used to be an immense garden megalopolis prior to the arrival of the conquistadors. The scientific community's estimates of the precolonial population in the Amazon rainforest vary widely, with the most daring ones approximating 100 million people.

Ridiculed and written off in the past by the international scientific community, many ancient spiritual perspectives are now being increasingly confirmed by cutting-edge research in various fields of study, including neuropsychology and quantum physics. Exciting as these discoveries may be, they provide merely circumstantial evidence. These findings represent a tiny glimpse into the evolutionary potential that the ancient civilizations embodied to a much greater degree than our current one. The inner life of those nearly forgotten civilizations is the real treasure depicted in the Peruvian legends of El Dorado and Paititi. All the external accomplishments of the ancient civilizations, including immense cities made of pure gold, such as El Dorado, were constructed in honor of the sacred geometry and symbolic meanings that far transcended any material riches.

In this book, I share my learnings from the first six months of my Amazonian healing journey as an essential introduction into the world of the ancients. I still regularly practice all of the tools in this book. Many people with whom I shared this wisdom over the years have also found it to be highly practical and beneficial.

For the past two decades, I have continued to study and consult with elders, Indigenous guides, ethnobotanists, anthropologists, and archaeologists of both the Peruvian Amazon and the Andes. The clues, revealed to me through these encounters as well as those discovered through personal practice, have been pieced together, thread by thread, to re-create the spiritual discipline of an almost-forgotten and highly advanced civilization. Many elders I met referred to their ancestral wisdom as *the Evolutionary Science of humanity.* Had I gone to the rainforest just a few years later, I'd likely not have had access to many of these teachings, since most of my teachers had left this plane of existence by that time.

I have since come to honor all the individuals who are living wisdom lineage carriers I encountered on my path of awakening as the embodied fragments of an entire primordial civilization—one with much to teach us today.

Nature Within, Nature Without

Over many years, I have worked with a number of people who long to embody their genuine nature and to walk through the trials of their life with greater strength and clarity—not just so they can live with a daily sense of purpose and meaning, but so they can be of benefit to others, especially amid the many compounding crises of our world.

I especially wrote this book for those who:

- Feel there is a greater purpose to life than what their mundane existence offers, and who wish to discover it through their own personal experience rather than hearsay

- Have had mind-blowing spiritual experiences in ceremony but without the objective guidance to integrate their experiences in a meaningful way

- Have been on intensive spiritual and plant medicine retreats and are in the process of integrating the insights they gained

- Are at a crossroads in their life (e.g., have a chronic illness, have been through major life changes, are in the process of questioning their path or redefining their purpose, etc.)

Beyond Ayahuasca encourages you to step into your own pristine nature: by helping you work with all the circumstances of your life (rather than escape them, which is often a reason people seek the spiritual path), come out of a defeatist mentality, take greater responsibility for your life, and apply an empowered perspective to all situations.

This book provides individual guidance for the transformation of consciousness. The particular rites of passage and initiations of one's life all relate to circumstances that are unique to each individual. *Beyond Ayahuasca* empowers you to transform your relationship to yourself and the Earth through a series of tools and practices, questions for self-inquiry and guided contemplation, reminders of the power to stay "real" and accountable throughout your spiritual journey, and information about the Evolutionary Science of humanity that will aid you in recognizing the beneficial and harmful patterns in your life.

Ayahuasca is becoming more of a household name, and people are looking for a deeper insight into the tradition, discipline, science behind it, and practical application in daily life. While Ayahuasca is an integral part of the ancient Amazonian culture, it is a tool to be utilized skillfully rather than the main focus. Although Ayahuasca first became famous in the West because of psychedelic culture, it was never intended for the purpose of generating hallucinogenic entertainment for the modern consumerist mindset. Furthermore, engaging Ayahuasca as a mind-training tool entails a rigorous process of cultivating insight into one's own consciousness in everyday life by facing all adversities with an open heart.

This book honors the cultural context of the traditions I have learned so much from while remaining applicable to our modern circumstances. Your individual engagement is fully invited, similar to a traditional Amazonian apprenticeship program. The purpose of evolutionary healing is awakening insight into your true nature, which relates to inner peace, unconditional love, and a synergistic connection between the mind and the heart. Storytelling is considered a medicine in itself in the Amazonian culture. Immersion in the story allows for spiritual practice to become a fluid experience.

Please note that this isn't about "mastering" the information in this book. It is not meant as a course to race through in order to receive some kind of spiritual certification or cross an "accomplishment" off your spiritual bucket list. It's not about the destination, but the journey; as such, this book is meant to be a lifetime tool. It's also a mirror for the inherent potential of each individual, guiding your whole existence to be a prayer or offering to the highest joy, which is continuously awakening to the infinite depths of love. This is what I learned from my teachers, and I hope this is what you will take from this book.

Unlike a retreat, where we step out of our habitual environment, this book is designed to help you create new habits within your daily environment and gradually resculpt your current habits and perspectives, such that you feel empowered to bravely face the circumstances of your life—and to transform your reality so that it mirrors your nature, which is already whole and complete.

While natural landscapes are diminishing all over the world, including in the Amazonian region, Indigenous living wisdom points out the indestructible nature within each being. Even in the most unnatural setting, we can remember who we are at our core.

The Organization of Your Journey

This book interweaves my journey of spiritual discovery with a deep dive into the ancient living cultures of the Amazon. Rather than presenting it as a typical prescriptive guide that takes you, the reader, along a path of spiritual progress, I have written it as an immersive mythical experience. Through storytelling and dialogue, it is my intention to transport you directly into the jungle where I first unearthed many primordial truths so that you can have an experience from a first-person perspective, as if you are going through the initiations and Indigenous rites of passage yourself, in the present time.

In sharing vulnerable aspects of my own journey, I hope to provide a mirror for your personal inquiry. The tools and reflection questions that are threaded throughout the chapters are designed to be simple yet profound; as you integrate these practices into your own life, you will discover that they are an extremely effective form of mind training that aims to demystify a seemingly exotic (and outlandish to the Western mind) Amazonian tradition, making it relevant to your modern life.

Throughout this book, you will also come into contact with the people I met along my spiritual path. The traditions I'd sought could not give me any ultimate answers . . . but they could point the way for the answers to be found within.

Although I studied with a Yahua elder and was adopted by the Yahua nation back in 2003, Don Sinchi, who is at the heart of the teachings I present, is a fictional "composite" character, informed by the many elders and teachers I met in the first several months of my journey. As I was guided by my teachers to bring the vast wisdom of the ancestors into a focal point, Don Sinchi has become an embodiment of all the evolved qualities I have witnessed in many Amazonian elders throughout the years. He is the Amazonian healer archetype representing the multitude of human qualities that form the mosaic of Evolutionary Science.

Over the years, I've seen how the Amazonian spiritual lineages are expressed through people who cultivate them to a profound degree. The more we seek to cultivate these enlightened qualities, the more likely it is that we'll find the peace, clarity, and well-being that the world today so direly needs.

This book is organized into two parts. Part 1 sets the stage for transformation and embodied realization. As you are introduced to the Amazon and the Indigenous elder Don Sinchi, you'll go on a corresponding journey through the maze of your own life experience that may be keeping you trapped in a state of spiritual amnesia—the disconnect from a natural state of awakened heart consciousness. My wish is that, as you follow along with my story and experiences, as well as the tools and reflections provided, you'll go through a profound clearing process of your own.

Part 1 sets the stage for Part 2 of the book. In stepping into your own journey through the book with the spirit of what Zen monk Shunryu Suzuki Roshi referred to as *beginner's mind,* you'll be introduced to a series of more specific practices that make up the Indigenous worldview. We'll dive into the meaning of interconnectedness, as well as the power of dreamwork. We'll also explore in greater depth the mythological realm of the Amazon, encompassing the plant and animal kingdoms. In addition, I'll touch upon key aspects of the traditional Indigenous perspective, including the importance of maintaining a sense of humor and not taking oneself too seriously in the midst of life's inevitable storms.

As I mentioned, the tools interspersed throughout each chapter are simple practices meant to deepen your experience and introduce you to the basic tenets of Amazonian Evolutionary Science in a clear and practical way. The reflection questions at the end of each chapter will help you further integrate your learning and keep an open, agile, curious heart as you engage in your own spiritual inquiry.

Three Pillars on the Path of Indigenous Ancestral Wisdom

Indigenous ancestral wisdom is at the heart of this book. According to the elders I studied with, the essence of the Amazonian tradition has always been about the ability of the human spirit to adapt to change, be curious, collaborate, and shine in the face of adversity.

All rituals, ceremonies, and rites of passage are the vessels that introduce that essence into our daily existence. Without the practical application of the meaning that specific symbols bring into our current existence, cultural appropriation by the consumerist mentality automatically takes place. The same rituals that were meant to help one get real with oneself can become another mask that keeps us from spiritual maturity.

For the Indigenous people of the rainforest, their immediate environment symbolizes the outer facets of the inner psyche. What happens when the modern world comes to them is that they are often unable to navigate the unfamiliar outer landscapes and consequently get lost in their inner ones. For example, not seeing the poisonous snakes in the corrupt mining and logging corporations invading their lands can lead to alcoholism, gambling, and crime in the younger generations of Amazonian people. The current predicament makes it necessary for the elders to reintroduce the same ancestral essence into a new world, in a way that keeps the essence relevant to the symbols of our current existence.

To bring the ancestral wisdom into your life in a pragmatic way that's relevant to your experience, it is necessary to build intercultural bridges that allow for deeper realization of ancestral states of consciousness. The ancestors engaged their minds through a poetic interplay of metaphors, symbols, and a dreamlike approach to daily life. In today's world, logical thinking prevails, but it's essential to awaken the more ancient part of the human brain for the journey of self-realization to be effective.

It's up to you to check the guidance of these lineages against your individual experience and recognize the universal principles that live beneath the appearance of the mundane. With selective hearing, it's easy to implement what is only advantageous to the monkey mind controlled by reactive impulses.

Let's look at the differences in each of our life experiences as a personal labyrinth each of us must figure out for ourselves. Although the life experiences forming that labyrinth may appear different on the surface, the range of feelings, emotions, and states are the same. The freedom of choice that can determine the way out of the maze depends on your willingness to face the emotional fabric that was responsible for the creation of the labyrinth in the first place.

To get the most out of reading, I encourage you to consider your own experiences of being out in the wilderness as a mirror for your own nature. For many millennia, the ambience of the Amazon, created by an immense diversity of flora and fauna, has been a perfect stage for the ancient mystery schools to initiate humans into our true potential.

Imagine yourself lost in the Amazon rainforest, wild animals shrieking on all sides, dense foliage obscuring every step. What kind of qualities could you cultivate to help you find your way? Obviously, panic, fear, frustration, resentment, or anger will only get you more lost. Being angry at the slowly approaching jaguar or taking it personally that he wants you for lunch will not help the situation, either.

Throughout this book, there are three pillars to keep in mind, which you'll be exploring in the teachings and practical exercises:

1. Understand the different unprocessed emotional energies that unconsciously determine the choices that have contributed to your everyday experiences ("getting lost in the jungle").

This is all about scouting your inner landscape and mapping the landmarks for both positive traits and disturbing afflictions. You may be surprised at how much these landmarks affect you without you even realizing it. Initially, it can be painful to open your eyes fully and grow increasingly aware of all those disempowering dynamics we often try so hard to ignore, pretending we aren't lost at all.

Even so, it's essential to come to terms with life's adversities, no matter how great or insignificant they may appear, in order to lay the groundwork and begin the journey home. This will become the steady ground under your feet that allows for sustainable progress.

The inner journey entails the recognition of circular patterns in your life—all the recurring challenges and disempowering relationships: with yourself first and foremost, and then with others.

2. The more you become familiar with the adversities and afflictions in your life and see the degree to which they're ingrained, the more clearly you can assess what your challenges are and what's required to overcome them.

This is when you start to develop a strategy for taking full responsibility for your own life. We're all directly responsible for perpetuating the disempowering impulsive reactions and negative habits that cause us to lose ourselves in the labyrinth of avoidance.

Developing a strategy and clearly seeing how to apply it against overwhelming odds requires developing a relationship with intensity. In the West, we often see intensity as something to be avoided. We can see this mentality at play when things don't go our way, or when we experience accidents or the sudden onset of disease, or when untamed natural forces cause disasters inside and out. In ancient traditions, however, intensity offers the opportunity to practice grounded presence, levelheadedness, and objectivity, because intensity is perceived as a conduit for remembering oneself as a channel of fearless love. Channeling that intensity in a creative, mindful way can help us focus our energy to face the adversities of life rather than run from them every time things don't go our way.

So, what will it take for us all to become mature, aware, and free human beings capable of finding our way through even the most complex and intense life circumstances and conditions? This takes us to step three.

3. While the first two steps prepared you to acknowledge and become aware of the task at hand, now you will uncover the spark of motivation significant enough to encourage continuous, sustained effort, which is essential on the journey of self-realization.

The essence of all the practices in this book is learning to maintain a continuous stream of heart-centered awareness throughout each moment of life. Obviously, maintaining such a conscious stream of awareness requires a sustained effort. That's where the motivational spark comes in.

In my case, it took continuous engagement and personal initiative involving a combination of insights, realizations, changes in lifestyle, and ancestral guidance that were relevant to my own journey. All of this helped me go into full remission from what is considered to be an incurable and often terminal genetic health condition within eight months of arriving in the Amazon rainforest. And yet, healing from that condition was just the beginning of a much deeper journey that continues to this day on subtler levels.

The real effort in the practical application of these tools isn't about forcing change, but becoming aware of all the aspects in your life of which you're currently unaware. Awareness itself becomes the natural catalyst for positive change and healing. It becomes the signposts along the way, as we reconnect with the metaphorical home our souls long to return to.

Happy trails as you do the important work of scouting your inner landscape!

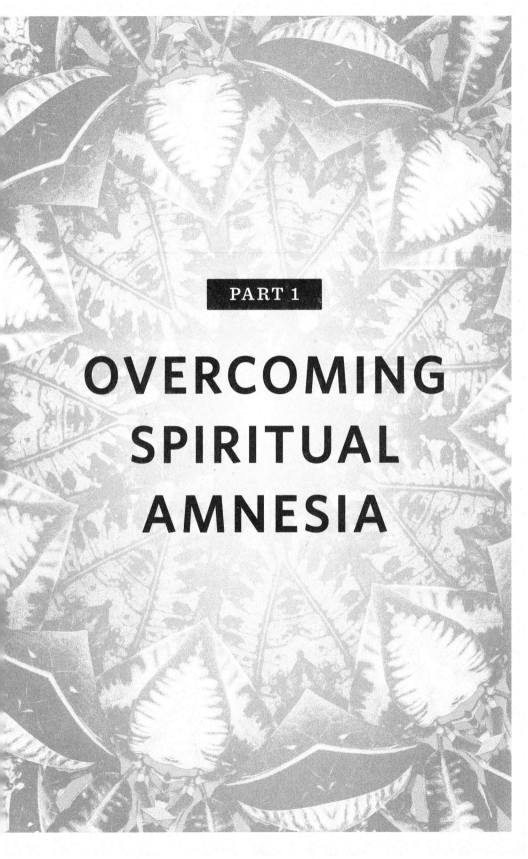

PART 1

OVERCOMING SPIRITUAL AMNESIA

CHAPTER 1

FROM SPIRITUAL AMNESIA TO ANCESTRAL WISDOM

The tribal chief looked meaningfully at me and put a finger to his mouth, signaling me to be quiet and listen. We sat with him, motionless, surrounded by the dense rainforest for a while. All of a sudden, a sense of extraordinary serenity overcame me. It was so tangible, I could almost grasp it with my hands.

The setting sun was slowly dimming the light of the green foliage surrounding us. The night birds awoke, greeting the slowly forming mantle of darkness with their lullabies. As the early evening turned to dusk, wisps of fog floating in the humid, tropical air became even more pronounced. The elder was about to impart wisdom of universal significance.

All of a sudden, out of the Indigenous elder's mouth an official announcement blasted, as if through a loudspeaker, and broke the enchantment of the mystical landscape. I found myself awakening in the airplane to the voice of the pilot over the loudspeaker: "We will be landing shortly in the Aeropuerto Internacional Francisco Secada Vignetta near the city of Iquitos."

I looked in disbelief around me. The dream I'd just had felt like a vivid premonition of what was to come. I was excited at the prospect of meeting a real-life representative of an ancient culture I had only encountered vague references to throughout my life. I was also quite anxious, as it was my first solo trip outside of my comfort zone in New York City—and I had no idea where to start once I landed in the vast territory of the Amazon rainforest. For the millionth time, I thought about what had brought me to undertake such an endeavor, against the sound advice of my family and friends.

The city of Iquitos, where I initially landed, was introduced to me as one of the main gateways into the Peruvian Amazon. A massive, bustling urban area with sparkling neon lights, noisy three-wheeled motorcar rickshaws, and clouds of pollution, it felt like a paradox in the midst of a region widely regarded as the lungs of the planet. One local told me there was even a Guinness world record bestowed upon Iquitos as the biggest, most isolated city in the world. The only way to get to it was by boat or plane. Surrounding the city were thousands of miles of pristine Amazon rainforest. Despite its isolated location, it seemed that Iquitos had ended up with some of the worst aspects of modern civilization.

After about two months of struggling to locate a healer to work with, I stumbled upon a block in my path. Many local curanderos did not seem to have the integrity of people in whose hands I could entrust my life. They were either drunkards or charlatans trying to get as much money as possible, using their charisma and "mystical" knowledge to attract and exploit desperate people. The locals I met referred to Ayahuasca as a commercial hallmark name for a sideshow attraction, rather than an integral element within a profound cultural context.

Seemingly, there was no longer a place for traditional healers in a society overrun with plastic, drugs, alcohol, pharmaceuticals, and industrialism. The "shamans" I had met, either in the city or its outskirts, were neither interested in the deeper values of humanity nor in the actualization of our inherent human potential. Some actually knew certain tricks that were a part of their shamanic trade and were busy exploiting the little knowledge they had. Ironically, they were the celebrity shamans of the Ayahuasca tourist industry, bent on achieving material "happiness," rather than caring for nature and people.

While there were obvious traces of spiritual, mystical, and healing traditions, there was also plenty of evidence pointing to the corruption and dilution of the ancient culture by modern society. Most of the local population seemed to be imitating Western society while belittling their own heritage. Ayahuasca was treated as a tourist extravaganza without any other practical value.

Thankfully, the homeless kids, called *piranhas* by the locals, were the first to show me there was more to the Amazonian culture than met the eye. These children were notorious for stealing from or selling drugs to foreigners, thus earning their "piranha" reputation. As soon as I mentioned Ayahuasca upon their approach to initiate a conversation, they immediately exhibited signs of fear, respect, and superstition.

I noticed by their behavior that they knew the power of Ayahuasca, not just by hearsay—and yet, despite already being used to a dangerous street life, they were terrified of it. The idea that tourist shows and *brujeria* (black witchcraft or sorcery) were all that remained of an ancient healing tradition left me feeling disillusioned.

It was not until I experienced the hopelessness of my situation that my luck began to shift. In my last attempt to find a genuine healer, I befriended a scout from the Bora tribe who agreed to take me on a two-week journey into the rainforest, visiting isolated Indigenous settlements along the way. It was a survival expedition, meaning we took no food or water with us. I wore a huge backpack with a lot of useless things stuffed inside, against the advice of my guide. Consequently, I got a chance to admit my ignorance with every step through the swampy trail. Cursing and swearing, I fell into every ditch and mud puddle along the way. I had only myself to blame.

Being at the mercy of the rainforest, I was also hungry a lot of the time. We ate only what my guide could catch and forage, which included wild nuts, fruits, slugs, frogs, and whatever else the rainforest offered us. On one occasion, we even ate a monkey. A big predator was about to have it for lunch, right when I unintentionally scared it off with my loud cursing and clumsy steps. I was concerned at how my sick GI tract would react to it all, and morally, I was not so keen on eating my Darwinian predecessor. The Bora guide laughed loudly at my repulsion. He explained that since I'd scared off the jaguar and he didn't come back to devour us, we should see his prey as an offering of the forest spirits and honor them by eating it. I agreed; somehow, my stomach did not object afterward. We also sipped slightly bitter water from special vines, which my guide knew how to identify. He explained to me that only some vines contain drinking water, and that water has many medicinal properties.

My friend also shared with me about the natives living in the surrounding areas, who, to this day, rarely come out of the rainforest. I began nagging him about finding a healer who lives deep in the rainforest among these people. He was initially reluctant, expressing that the healers today are not the same as they used to be. Wet and muddy, I insisted and my friend acquiesced.

The few small settlements we passed through had no healers of their own. However, people in the last settlement pointed us to a distant, solitary dwelling of one healer my guide was also familiar with. When we finally arrived at the dilapidated dwelling of the healer, we found him drunk and belligerent, which only enhanced my sense of futility.

Toward the completion of that intense and exhausting expedition, I had a chance meeting with a local elderly woman named Sacha. She worked in the regional municipality and was sent to evaluate a tourist lodge that my guide and I visited on our final day of the expedition. She shared that her name meant "forest" in the native intertribal language of Kichwa and that she was a mestizo, with both Spanish and Indigenous blood.

Sacha was intrigued by the ancient culture of the region and throughout the years had befriended many native healers in the surrounding areas. Although her main passion was social anthropology, Sacha rarely took part in the sacred Indigenous ceremonies. Nevertheless, she agreed to introduce me to an old friend from the Yahua tribe who was one of the very few she trusted with her life. Sacha shared with me that he was a tribal chief and a wondrous healer who lived quite a distance from Iquitos. My hope of encountering a real, trustworthy healer was reignited.

The Cataclysm of the Ancient Amazonian Society

After a week of recovery due to the intense wilderness excursion, we met with Sacha on a Sunday morning when she was off work. She hailed a local "moto-taxi" that drove us to the busy river port of Bellavista Nanay, from where we set sail on our journey. The boat we were in, huddled among many locals traveling with live chickens, ducks, and small farm animals, was called a *peke-peke*. Sacha told me it was named after the very slow motor that makes pecking noises.

The voyage along the snakelike river, immersed in the lush green canopy of the rainforest, became more enjoyable. The songs of exotic birds could be heard through the reverberating hum of the peke-peke. Occasionally, Sacha would point out the shapes of gray dolphins in the distance, rising above the water line. They seemed reluctant to come closer to us and the strange, noisy contraption we were in. The fact that I was actually in the legendary Amazon basin began to dawn on me. Out of curiosity, I asked Sacha if she knew the history of the region, and specifically, the origin of the name *Iquitos*.

What I learned from Sacha was important context—and it changed the disgust and disillusionment that had informed my journey thus far.

The first official settlers of the region were an Indigenous group who called themselves *Iquito*. The city of Iquitos was built on a semi-island resembling the shape of a turtle, immersed in the Amazon River. The creation myths of the Iquito tribe spoke of a gigantic turtle traversing the length of the river; the turtle had decided to take a nap in the location where the city stands today. The elders of that tribe had a prophecy that the turtle would nap for many millennia. One day, however, it would awaken to fulfill its journey back to the great ocean.

Even though that tribe was among the first to be wiped out by the conquistadors, it lived on in the city's name. To this day, all the inhabitants of the local Loreto region are called *Charapas*, an ancient name for a turtle species that is still alive today. Some elders say that the spirit of the Iquito tribe lives on in all the people of modern Iquitos, slowly awakening the Charapas to fulfill that ancient prophecy by remembering to honor Mother Nature.

I thought to myself that with all the pollution and squalor I'd witnessed in Iquitos, the "awakening" was happening a little too slowly. But as I learned over time, the current state of affairs in the region had not simply occurred in a vacuum.

Many of us in the West are only vaguely familiar with the rich histories of other regions of the world—particularly those we've been taught to view as the Third World. My disgust toward what I saw in Iquitos was softened as I came into a deeper awareness of the history of the Amazonian people.

The appearance of the first Western explorers and missionaries, alongside Francisco de Orellana in the 15th century, announced the end of an era for the people of the region. Prior to that, the tribes of the Amazon were rarely physically sick. The first explorers came from overpopulated European cities filled with pestilence and disease. Upon first contact with Indigenous culture, these explorers compared the natives to godlike beings for their incredible vitality.

When the smallpox pandemic began ravaging the Amazon, the Indigenous elders knew the foreigners had brought this curse, yet they did not blame them for it. Instead, they perceived the source of the illness to be the collective degradation of human values that had taken over the planet.

The people here had also been afflicted by the same plague of spiritual amnesia, which is the loss of heart-centered values, resulting in greed, aggression, fear, and pride, among other toxic qualities. However, the people of the Amazon were affected to a much lesser extent due to their isolation from the rest of the world. The wise elders encouraged people to stay connected with the wisdom of Mother Nature. But, as history shows, the demise of so many ancient civilizations that had a stronger connection to nature was sadly inevitable, especially as "exploration" became more routine and the world grew smaller.

The sickness of humanity began to mutate into physical disease. As a result, 95 percent of the pre-Columbian Amazonian population was wiped out, and innumerable human lives were extinguished over a very short period of time.

It was one of the greatest cataclysms in human history that few people know about today. In a strange twist of fate, the very same explorers who unwittingly waged biological warfare on the Amazonian people chronicled in their personal diaries the splendors of a mysterious civilization that they had "discovered." Sadly, these explorers were the first and last external witnesses of that ancient culture when it was still intact. Their records detailed a magnificent kingdom with an immense population living in profound communion with nature.

The accounts of the first explorers spoke not of ignorant savages, living like animals in a primitive milieu, but rather, painted a completely different picture of the world: human dwellings straight from a fantasy world, with entire cities made of towers constructed on and between colossal ancient trees. Since no Westerner had ever found anything remotely resembling those initial discoveries, they were discredited for a long time as made-up fables. Only recently, archaeological discoveries have verified the accounts of the first European arrivals.

Ironically, the initial clues about the groundbreaking findings came from the aerial photos of deforested regions of the Amazon. Kept hidden for centuries under the thick canopy of the rainforest were ancient paved roads that spanned thousands of kilometers. In addition, moats and aqueduct channels of precise geometrical shapes surrounded ancient cities. The Amazonian ancestors also left behind mounds of great agricultural productivity. An immense population was sustained with an abundance of nutrient-dense food amid what's known today to be a desert. Ancient terra preta soil technology was found, based on advanced microbiology and biochemistry. (*Terra preta* refers to a fertile soil that is purposely made by combining charcoal, ash, and organic waste.) Modern science is unable to replicate the effects of terra preta to this day.

What Sacha shared with me was extremely powerful. Not only did the pre-Columbian people live in absolute abundance, but also they were able to do so in a sustainable way—regenerating rather than decimating their natural resources. The ancient ways were in stark contrast to the extractive values of the conquistadors.

Currently, the Indigenous population of the Amazon basin is a tiny percentage of what existed prior to European contact. Although far lesser in number, the inhabitants of this region live in extreme poverty today. Sadly, having lost a connection to their ancestral way of life through contact with the conquistadors, Amazonian people now continuously overexploit their environment. They leave a wake of destruction and desertification in place of an old-growth rainforest, just to buy imported foods necessary for their survival.

I understood from my conversation with Sacha that much had happened since the world of the Amazonian people had fallen apart with the arrival of the conquistadors. It was devastating to recognize that what was around me was a distant echo of the Indigenous people's ancestral glory.

Sacha was taking me to see a Yahua elder. She told me that the Yahuas had been among the first to make contact with the Europeans. They had also been integrating their ancestral wisdom into Western society longer than any other Amazonian tribe. Because of the Yahua chief's familiarity with the modern mindset, he was now helping many people from the city of Iquitos to heal from physical and emotional maladies by sharing the wisdom of the Amazonian ancestors.

I thought to myself that the story of the Amazon was one that still echoes throughout the world and is unfortunately not an isolated case. Instead, it is becoming the norm. It is the consequence of a system that has overtaken the world, and that relentlessly commodifies and objectifies nature. Similarly, the Jordanian desert was once a lush rainforest. Large parts of Australia, northern Africa, and more recently, the island of Madagascar all serve as pertinent warnings about the destruction of nature by our fellow humans. In fact, the issues plaguing the world today are symptoms of collective spiritual amnesia overtaking humankind.

Arriving at a Genuine Connection

It was already dark as our peke-peke boat slowly glided across the river Tahuayo, approaching the remote Indigenous settlement of the lower Amazon basin. I became struck by the sight of numerous candles and oil lamps shimmering inside wide-open huts. The dwellings, edging on the riverside, were perched atop wooden poles in case of flooding. With no walls, the houses were embellished with woven palm leaves for roofs. The village was exactly how I'd imagined the fantasy worlds of my childhood books: a mystical place where magic surely dwelled.

Since we had gotten to be good friends through our mutual fascination with ancient cultures, Sacha was keen on accompanying me to her friend. She told me that he was a well-known *Rimyurá*, which is the Yahua term for a chief and a medicine man.

The monotonous rambling of the boat's motor suddenly stopped, and Sacha leaned toward me intently. "Nobody knows we're coming," she said, "but let's hope Don Sinchi is around—he's known to go on forays in the woods to collect herbs for days, or sometimes even weeks at a time!"

As soon as we disembarked, we were immediately greeted by a tall, young Indigenous man who stood in the dark shadow of a nearby tree. He was practically invisible, veiled by the night, and startled us when he came into the dim moonlight. He introduced himself as Chispa and told us in broken Spanish to follow him to Rimyurá Sinchi's house. Apparently, he had been informed by Don Sinchi that two people matching our exact description were about to arrive and should be escorted to the Rimyurá straight away.

Sacha and I looked at each other, perplexed—she had just told me that nobody knew of us coming!

We followed the man into the night, venturing deeper into the forest's soundscapes for an hour and a half. Finally, we reached a small clearing in the nearly impenetrable fortress of trees, where a solitary house stood. The house, unlike the dwellings by the river, was not on stilts and had wooden boards for walls.

Without pausing or announcing ourselves, we followed Chispa and entered the simple dwelling. Right away, my attention was drawn like a magnet toward an elderly man sitting on a small wooden bench by the opposite wall from the entrance. He appeared to be in his 70s; somehow, just seeing him made my mind settle. Harmony and calmness emanated from his presence. He had chiseled facial features and brilliant, wide-open eyes that penetrated the object of his focus.

After a long yet comforting pause, the elder walked over to us with wide-open arms, embracing us like long-lost companions.

"We were waiting for your arrival to start dinner," he said, smiling. Noticing our bemused expressions, he added with delight, "Last night in a ceremony, the spirits informed me of your impending arrival—great timing, too!" He introduced himself as Don Sinchi. With tangible excitement and a twinkle in his eyes, the elder then turned toward the dinner table and said, "You must be hungry after such a long journey. Come, please join me for a delicious meal!"

We headed over to his table, where a local dish known as *patarashka* was already set at each of our places. Still steaming, our platters consisted of piranha fish wrapped in banana leaves prepared over a *tushpa*. The tushpa is another ancient Amazonian novelty that consists of an elevated table filled with earth and a grill placed over it, eliminating the need to cook on the ground with a bent back.

After being serenaded by the cicadas at our candlelit dinner, I volunteered to help Don Sinchi fill water buckets in a nearby creek for use in the kitchen. It was a 20-minute walk beneath the dim light of the moon, and I kept stumbling, trying to catch up to the elder. Don Sinchi was so limber in his gait that it appeared as though our roles had been reversed. I acted like a clumsy old man, while the Yahua chief exhibited the prowess of a young tribal warrior.

Once we got to the creek, the youthful elder invited me to sit down and enjoy the moment. Under the massive trees looming over us, I unwittingly sank into a state of deep restfulness. My thoughts trickled away, following the sound of the small creek. I was enamored with my new environment.

After all the negative experiences I'd had with healers up until then, I occasionally glanced critically at the Yahua elder. I wondered whether he was going to be just like all the other "shamans" I met, despite my positive first impression.

All of a sudden, the Rimyurá broke his silence and started talking. "I see you being intuitively drawn here, burdened by many questions. You've come this far seeking the same answers that humanity has pondered from the time of its conception: What is the purpose of life? Who are we?" He suddenly paused, seeing my perplexed expression.

I smiled sheepishly and asked if he knew the answers. What he shared with me was the wisdom of the ancestors that has been preserved in great secrecy over generations, under severe persecution for all who carried it. This information would ultimately change my life.

The Primary Purpose of All Life-Forms

Myth and storytelling are known to be powerful medicines in many Indigenous tribes, and this was especially true among the Yahua.

Don Sinchi told me a legendary tale, which he described as never-ending and with no beginning. It spoke of his wisdom lineage, which would go on living even after the Yahua nation ceased to exist: "The basic creation story of the Yahuas stems from the Great Primordial Heavenly Spirit known as Grandfather Jarichu, who created the complementary opposites that sustain our world. The Yahuas believe that the divine union of universal forces in nature is the creative source of all life. The lives of all of Earth's inhabitants are sustained by an intimate relationship that Mother Earth (Mokane) is having with Father Sun (Eñu).

"Our reality is filled to the brim with ordinary miracles, which most people today take for granted, such as rain falling from the sky. In the Yahua tribe, the sun and the Earth are seen as embodied expressions of higher consciousness and unconditional love. The raindrops falling from the sky are the semen of Father Sun impregnating Mother Earth.

"According to Indigenous wisdom, this divine love affair between the heart of creation and her higher consciousness is the origin of all life-forms in the universe. All beings are the children of the Great Spirit of Love, known as *Munaychi* in the intertribal Kichwa language. The Great Father and the Great Mother are here to continuously remind us of our own inherent potential to merge the mind and heart as one."

I contemplated Don Sinchi's words. As I was starting to learn, finding a way to be a clear channel of boundless love was the core teaching of Evolutionary Science, as Don Sinchi referred to it. Although I had come to the path primarily for the sake of personal healing—and in an act of renunciation of my former life, which had brought only pain and disappointment—Don Sinchi was helping me see that any spiritual training was for the purpose of gradually remembering how to channel infinite amounts of love.

"Don Sinchi, what about all the other feelings and experiences that are *not* love?" I couldn't help but interject.

Don Sinchi smiled mischievously and said, "There's nothing else but love, and yet, it's your journey of evolution to realize that everything you judge and label as 'not' love is based on not knowing any better . . . In nature, there's only love, but when it's not imbued with the light of consciousness, it becomes destructive, rather than creative. Consciousness without the heart is cruel, and good intentions without discernment pave the road to hell. This energy of love that we are all born as channels of is not some kind of mystical energy to fantasize about. It's the energy of each moment that is unlike any other moment before it."

The elder peered at me as I swatted mosquitoes and added with a smile, "Are you open to each new moment of your life, despite all of the disturbing mosquitoes, circumstances, sensations, and emotions?"

"Sometimes I'm open, and sometimes I'd rather not be present with what bothers me," I admitted. "That's when I distract myself from the discomfort that a stressful experience brings."

"Yes, that's how the plague of forgetfulness works—avoiding life, numbing out, and having lots of preconceived notions about how the world should revolve around you," Don Sinchi said with a kind smile. "However, the constantly changing nature of reality contradicts that mistaken view, which results in constant anxiety based on avoidance and clinging. The way out of that vicious cycle is to realize that true happiness is intertwined with the fearless wisdom of the heart.

"Lasting, timeless joy is only possible when we no longer depend on conditions that are nice and comfortable, but fully trust in the capacity to consciously remain open and at ease in each moment, no matter what. The journey of remembrance starts with catching ourselves whenever we forget to remain open. The more we see our forgetfulness, the more we can remember to keep opening to the endless diversity of life experience. Now, don't you start feeling bad about habitually disconnecting from being alive. Beating yourself up about not being open will only make you shut down more. Practice makes perfect!"

The elder smiled kindly at me. His instructions reminded me of a saying I'd heard from a Zen practitioner once: *The master failed more than the student had ever tried.*

Suddenly, a mosquito bit me and I momentarily became distracted again. I looked at the Yahua elder to see how he dealt with the little buggers and then noticed that although we were sitting next to each other, the mosquitoes seemed to be attracted only to me. Don Sinchi was so at ease and emanated such well-being that a natural aura of protection prevented mosquitoes from biting him. I, on the other hand, was constantly fidgeting, fending off the insects, only to make them more curious about the taste of my blood. I tried not to react to the mosquitoes, seeing how my reactions only made me more irritated. Gathering myself, I asked, "What happens when someone completely forgets their original purpose as a living organism, Don Sinchi?"

The elder responded matter-of-factly: "Then, Universal Love ceases to be channeled harmoniously and creates an imbalance, or a dis-ease. The division and duality in the world today are the cause of so much suffering because we have collectively forgotten ourselves as channels of divine glory. Instead, humankind has turned into a self-absorbed soap opera."

I understood all too well, from my own experiences. I had already seen the way that I and others avoided life, numbed out, and built mental bulwarks against reality. Contemplating what Don

Sinchi had just shared, I realized that the journey of remembrance begins when we start to catch ourselves in every moment of forgetting to remain open. There were times prior to my coming to the Amazon when I found myself driving home without being conscious of where I was going or what I was doing, or when I zoned out of a conversation because I felt bored and uncomfortable, or when I started to multitask and lost track of my initial intention. Even during my time with Don Sinchi, I had experiences of fending off potential bug attacks to the degree that I was unable to enjoy the beauty of my surroundings. But the more I spent time with Don Sinchi, the more I began to realize it was possible to remember to keep opening to the endless diversity of life experiences.

At this stage, I was beginning to see that this diversity—even when I experienced pain, mental dullness, or in my case with the mosquitoes, discomfort—was life's way of helping me attune to the love that is at the very core of human nature.

Tool: Understanding and Working with Spiritual Amnesia

How do we begin to move out of our spiritual amnesia and back into our nature as conduits of Universal Love? A good practice to incorporate remembering into your life is to check throughout the day whether your decisions and actions arise from a place of love or of fear. Catch yourself when it's the latter; refuse to go along with unconscious habitual tendencies that developed over time. When we catch ourselves in the moment of decision-making with kindness and not self-judgment, we gradually dispel habitual tendencies and integrate conscious awareness into our every action. Nowadays, there are even mindful bell apps that ring at random times and can be used to help us check in with ourselves with greater intention and presence, until at some point, we can do this without any reminders.

Another way to dispel the effects of spiritual amnesia is to train yourself to lean in to discomfort. This is like shining a penetrating light through the thick fog of illusions that permeates our reality. While in the beginning, it may not necessarily feel like spirit is shining in the face of adversity, it is important to learn to rest with what bothers you. Even taking an extra breath or two when it feels unbearable, without running toward instant gratification or an escape, is already good progress on the path of remembrance.

Be at ease with what is, whatever it is has been a useful chant/prayer/mantra in my life to help me remember how to step out of hectic, reactive behavior, which always gets me in trouble!

REFLECTIONS

- One of my first great lessons on this spiritual journey was something that was ingrained in me as Don Sinchi told the creation myth. This lesson is that the primary purpose of all life-forms is to be essential links of love between our cosmic parents—the Mother and the Father, the material and the spiritual, the mind and the heart. We can do so by channeling love steadily and consciously throughout our life for the benefit of all. *What is your general experience of love?*

- For most people, love is deeply personal and connected to the people and situations that are intimately familiar to us. However, the greatest love in the universe is not the relational love most of us think of, which is usually more like the Buddhist concept of attachment, grasping, or clinging—referring to our tendency to cling to people and situations in the hope that they'll offer us lasting happiness or security. In contrast, Universal Love extends beyond the desire to be safe, comfortable, and in control. Rather, it is transcendent and impersonal—a love without pity through which one awakens to the heart's indestructible wisdom. *What was a time in your life when you experienced the flow of Universal Love, free of attachment or the desire for security?*

- There is a marvelous paradox at the heart of the spiritual journey. Even when we experience emotional states such as rage, jealousy, hatred, and anything else that feels like a far cry from love, there is only one ultimate truth: There is nothing but love. *Have you ever had the experience of intense, non-loving emotions eventually bringing you back to love, or of realizing the omnipresence of love in the middle of a difficult challenge? Have the circumstances of your life given way to the realization that there is nothing but love?*

- As soon as something troubles us, we shut down. The fight-flight-freeze response kicks in, and we find a way to avoid being with our experience. Often, especially in the West, we distract ourselves from the discomfort that stressful experiences bring, choosing, instead, to immerse ourselves in things like social media, online shopping, or attending to the growing list of items on our to-do list. Our lives have become increasingly "busy," but much of that busyness is wasted on avoidance instead of on developing the clear faculties that will help us realize our primary purpose: love. It may seem harmless enough. Many of us, even those of us on a path of consciousness, might say, "I can't deal with these feelings now, but I'll deal with them later." There's a domino effect to such a decision, and it leads to the collapse of our awareness. The more we leave the work of facing our feelings, our problems, our life, exactly as it is, for a "later" date, the more we forget how to live. *What is something in your life that you are avoiding out of fear? What is one simple action you can take to lean in to the discomfort with love and curiosity?*

CHAPTER 2

UNLOCKING THE EVOLUTIONARY SCIENCE

During my time with Don Sinchi, I learned that although spiritual amnesia had shrouded humanity in a fog of false ideas about who we are and where we come from, greater truths had once permeated the land. From all that Don Sinchi had shared, there was a time long before the advent of what we call "human history" when people lived in harmony with themselves, one another, and the planet as a whole. I thought of my own illness, and how living in such an imbalanced world—overrun by greed, consumerism, and violence—has the potential to create disease.

Only a few hours had passed since I first met Don Sinchi, but in some ways, it felt like centuries. As we sat by the creek near Don Sinchi's hut after our delicious dinner, getting ready to carry buckets of water to the elder's kitchen, I continued my conversation with him. "Don Sinchi, you mentioned that when Universal Love ceased to flow harmoniously and humans lost their way, dis-ease and imbalance came to be. Can you say more about that?"

He nodded. "The inevitable outcome of such a scenario is an imbalance within an organism. If ignored long enough, it manifests as either an internal illness or an outer misfortune. All the wars, natural disasters, and pandemics are direct consequences of our entire global population being out of whack.

"Yet, it's not a collective punishment, as some tend to see it. Our ancestral wisdom reminds us to recognize all of life's adversities as wake-up calls. Each of us becomes part of the resolution by remembering the shared heart of humanity as the main guiding force of our lives. Unity in diversity is the only way for all of us to live healthily, sustainably, and regeneratively. Outer change must be born from within.

"Our perspective is by no means unique in this recognition of humanity's basic predicament and its resolution. Over the years, I've met people from many spiritual traditions who all share this view. Sad as it sounds, such is our reality today, the evidence for which is omnipresent: humankind has lost its path, and the only way to find it again is by clearly seeing where we are heading as a collective, and why. The Evolutionary Science of our ancestors is key to remembering the potential of human aliveness on the innermost level, through all the hurdles of life."

Don Sinchi quieted down again. He seemed relaxed, yet fully alert and receptive to every sound within our environment. Noticing how at home he was in the rainforest, I followed the elder's cue and tried to meditate on the harmony of the sights, smells, and sounds surrounding us. I tried for what seemed like a long time, yet only had partial success. The story of humanity's demise and the mosquitoes continued to trouble me.

I shared with Don Sinchi how sad it had been for me to witness life on our planet being systematically drained and destroyed. The Rimyurá listened to me as he nodded.

"Yes, all those examples of nature being destroyed around the world are direct aftermaths of humanity's loss of culture. All the misfortunes in the world are caused by the mother of all diseases—the plague of forgetfulness. During the Amazonian cataclysm of the fifteenth century, our people tried to preserve their ancestral wisdom, since it was their most sacred treasure. In turn, that very wisdom allowed the survival of those few who truly embodied it."

Don Sinchi shared that the when humans began to lose their original culture of Universal Love, and to forget their higher purpose, humanity was faced with three choices:

1. **To degrade one's consciousness in order to survive:** The majority of the world's population today has chosen this option—lost in consumerism and instant gratification, and succumbing to a false sense of security and comfort at the expense of all that is sacred. As Don Sinchi shared, descending into our instinctual animalistic behavior, which is hardwired into our survival, while abandoning our human values, is the easiest of the three options to choose in the moment. However, it is always followed by grave long-term consequences.

2. **To perish physically but not degrade spiritually:** Don Sinchi explained that many of his ancestors had chosen this path, because their life circumstances no longer allowed for noble values to be cultivated and they were not willing to compromise their values by turning into vicious animals for the sake of survival.

3. **To evolve and thrive, both physically and spiritually:** This is the most harmonious choice we can make, but it is the path least trodden by humanity as a whole. In order to be successful at this, we must remember how to embody heart-centered awareness. This can be challenging, but it is the most beneficial and sustainable thing we can do for all of life on this planet. It is the path back to remembrance of our true origins, our true culture that we have been bereft of for so long. Many of us may be burdened by external and internal factors that can make life very difficult, such that we may feel as if we are under constant attack. However, if we apply Evolutionary Science to the fullest, we can find constructive ways to navigate hardship and remain attuned to our true nature.

I wondered aloud how we could choose physical and spiritual evolution, especially if the examples around us were by and large of degradation. It was no secret that spiritual amnesia seemed to be rendering many of our human efforts moot or fruitless. I knew all too well that even spiritual communities dealt with problems that could sometimes lead to decisions that lacked integrity.

When I asked Don Sinchi this, he remained quiet for a long moment, eyes closed, and then began speaking. "We must connect with the enlightened ancestors in order to forge a path for ourselves."

"How do we do that?" I asked.

With a stern expression, he said, "Though there are many prophecies left to us from the primordial times, before humans declared war on this planet and themselves, they all have one thing in common. They all draw their origin from the time of enlightened ancestors, a time when humanity was free from suffering. There are many tribes here in the Amazon, all reminiscing about a time when our planet was revolving around two suns."

Don Sinchi continued, and as our conversation deepened, I felt myself being transported to a time before time, when the legends of the ancestors were woven into people's daily reality and the recorded chronicles of modern society were yet to be written, while greater wisdom permeated the world.

The Enlightened Ancestors

Don Sinchi explained, "As hard as it may be for people nowadays to believe, once upon a time, people of the world experienced a continuous state of love and harmony in peaceful communion with all of life. The legends state that while humanity was anchored in the boundless wisdom of the heart, there was no such thing as dis-ease. There was also no one to heal, because everyone was always healthy. Not knowing anything apart from a heart-centered state of being, people had no need for any traditions, rituals, or medicines. They were ceaselessly nourished by Nature's all-encompassing, majestic love, and experienced every moment of life to be deeply healing.

"As time went on, humanity slowly began to forget love as the highest purpose. The greater the collective amnesia got, the more suffering became unleashed on the world. As a consequence of people's innate connection with nature becoming severed, the delicate balance of all life on our planet also became increasingly disturbed. After all, human civilization, with its cement jungles for cities and polluting technologies invading us today, began as an idea in people's heads. The 'progress' of modernity is just as ephemeral as this rainforest fog if it's destroying the delicate balance of life on this planet . . . and eventually, itself."

Seeing my awestruck reaction, he added, "Modern society is so proud of their moon landing, but our ancestors visited the moon first, eons ago. They even left their bare footprints on the moon's surface!"

I responded that I remembered hearing an urban legend as a kid about one of the first astronauts to step on the moon's surface, who claimed to have seen a bare human footprint that no one could explain.

Don Sinchi smiled, nodding in confirmation, and continued: "Just as many traditions have charted humanity's fall from grace through myths that delineated both missteps and redemption, the Amazonian legends also provided similar explanations for the dis-ease of collective spiritual amnesia . . . for our departure from love as our primary purpose. Some legends mention that humanity's fall from grace coincided with one of the two suns that the Earth used to orbit, when it spiraled away into another galaxy."

He went on to explain that it was during that legendary period that the vast majority of those who remembered themselves as love crossed into another realm of existence altogether. In that otherworldly realm, they were able to maintain a state of consciousness that the pandemic of forgetfulness could not touch. Spirit portals into that realm of enlightened ancestors were opened across the planet with a series of powerful ceremonies, unifying the intentions of millions of people. This region of the Amazon was one of them. There were reports of the conquistadors describing Spanish soldiers entering completely abandoned, empty settlements with no one for miles around and food still cooking on the stoves. Don

Sinchi noted that his people referred to the portal in this region as *Paititi*, a name originating from an ancient pre-Inca civilization—the Tiahuanacu culture. The original meaning of the word *Paititi* translates to "the heart of all hearts" or "the greatest treasure a heart can desire." (It was also the namesake for the Paititi Institute for the Preservation of the Environment and Indigenous Culture, which I co-founded as part of my commitment to embodying the awakened spirit of the individual through which planetary transformation is possible.)

The second interpretation of *Paititi* was especially misleading to many of the colonial explorers, whose hearts only knew greed for material possessions. For the Indigenous people, however, the greatest treasure was the ancient heritage of infinite human potential.

Don Sinchi said, "After the mass exodus of the ancients, a few of the enlightened ancestors stayed behind, to help all those who got trapped in the limbo of oblivion. These noble souls remained here on Earth just long enough to initiate lineages of living wisdom as reminders of who we all really are. This was the greatest of all treasures entrusted to us by those lineages—an energetic blueprint for the realization of infinite human potential. Only by rekindling humanity's primordial wisdom again and again can future generations be resuscitated from a spiritual coma amid the most severe global crisis that is yet to come."

I looked at Don Sinchi with some confusion. I understood that there were prophecies across spiritual and religious traditions that point to a catastrophic event with the power to break or remake humanity in a new light. I wondered if this was what he meant.

He seemed to read my mind. "At the end of the enlightened era here in the rainforest, all the tribes still lived in harmony, guided by the very last of the remaining enlightened ancestors. The legendary spiritual forefather of our ancestral wisdom is still revered throughout the rainforest today by different names, like Shapuinguito, Shapi Shiko, or Yoshin Tayta. The legends say that he lived for thousands of years and was wise beyond measure. All of the tribes regarded him as their great chief and a medicine man of such magnitude that he could heal people with a blink of an eye.

"Shapuinguito was an exceedingly just and compassionate being of light. Inevitably, though, the day came when he foresaw a new era of greater darkness approaching the Earth. The benevolent king was very sad for his fellow humans, who kept forgetting themselves as conduits of Universal Love. He also knew then that his time on this planet was coming to an end, leaving him no choice but to continue his evolutionary journey beyond the stars. Summoning his closest friends, he informed them that, being the last of his kind, it was time for him to leave his earthly shell behind and join the rest of his people.

"The great king left behind one magical forest being, who was his apprentice to keep helping our Yahua people; his name is Mayantu, and we still receive his healing help and guidance to this day. Before departing, Shapuinguito foretold the time when ignorance and confusion would reach a boiling point all over the world. He said it would be the darkest hour right before the dawn. Our enlightened ancestor revealed to us that it was all part of our universal parents' divine plan for catalyzing human evolution.

"Shapuinguito's last instructions for his closest student were to bury his body in a specific location and wait for two sacred plants to grow on his tombstone. Alchemically merging these two plants together in a particular way would allow ordinary people to access the dimension of Paititi. Because Paititi was his final destination, he could be contacted there with the help of these sacred plants. People who could reach that sacred dimension would then get the same healing and wisdom they were getting from Shapuinguito when he was alive on Earth. More so, the great healer said that those two plants would only be effective when engaged skillfully, the way his closest apprentices were taught. Without his instructions, it would be futile to navigate the infinitely vast ocean of the Great Spirit to the realm of enlightened ancestors—a place where there is no time, and everything is known."

Don Sinchi said that Shapuinguito, the last enlightened being of the rainforest, mentioned prior to his departure that although he was the last of his kind, there used to be many others like him, who'd also stayed behind all across the planet. I recognized that this concept was similar to the Mahayana Buddhist ideal of the *bodhisattva*, someone who reaches enlightenment but delays leaving this earthly plane out of the compassionate desire to guide other suffering beings to their salvation. And perhaps it is no different from accounts of light beings and ascended masters who come to our planet in order to plant the seeds of liberation in hearts that ache for more than the push-and-pull between desire and aversion, which inevitably leads to suffering. I wondered whether these ancient enlightened beings Don Sinchi was talking about had been in communication with one another with respect to how they could bring Universal Love back into human consciousness.

Don Sinchi explained that the last of the enlightened ancestors foresaw with great precision all the crucial evolutionary thresholds of humanity throughout time. Using clairvoyance, they collaborated on co-founding the lineages of living wisdom to keep the higher potential of humanity alive as a reminder to subsequent generations of humans. Different lineages across the world were designed to make distinct teachings and tools available at the right times, in ways that would be the most relevant to the collective evolutionary journey. Over time, these instructions were turned into the various spiritual traditions that are practiced today around the world. All of them had once been directly relevant to humanity's original heritage and birthright, but eventually, spiritual amnesia brought dogma into the original wellsprings of living wisdom. As the teachings became concretized into specific "rules" and instructions, the direct experience of divine union that was so essential for the enlightened ancestors was eroded until it became practically absent.

I was curious about how the different lineages of the world could join together in a single stream of wisdom to awaken our human potential. It seemed to me that humans were too busy attempting to one-up each other to prove that their gods and traditions were more legitimate than anyone else's. Understandably, many people in the secular West have a desire for connection with the sacred, but they are simultaneously disillusioned by the various "holy wars" that tend to obscure the bigger question: Can we, as one humanity, boldly step into our birthright of Universal Love to create a more harmonious world?

Don Sinchi responded, "Another prophecy of Shapuinguito is meant to be fulfilled when humanity reaches its darkest hour, when unseen chaos will run amok in people's hearts. It will be during that time that the remaining ancestral lineages from all over the world will reunite, guiding humanity home to the original heaven on Earth. Our ancestral lineage will have an essential role in the final merger of planetary wisdom."

As Don Sinchi shared, the Amazonian ancestral lineage is especially supported by nature's capacity to bridge the practical with the spiritual. In the Amazon, human beings' relationship with their true nature is made tangible. Mother Nature is the most evolved expression of Universal Love and consciousness, weaving the tapestry of life through all beings. According to Don Sinchi, Mother Nature's evolutionary love is exponential because all life-forms hold her creative essence. Indeed, life on this planet is a tiny expression of her vast potential, which extends into the farthest corners of the universe.

I remembered what the elder said about Shapuinguito's instructions to bury his body in a location where two plants would grow. "Don Sinchi, can you say more about the two plants you mentioned?"

He smiled. "Because ours is a wisdom lineage of direct experience, the two plants are mentioned in the prophecy as skillful instruments to help us fully face ourselves and remember our heritage as star beings, just like the enlightened ancestors who traversed the universe with the power of their consciousness."

Don Sinchi explained what this meant. His great-grandfather, a powerful healer who was also the chief of the Yahua tribe, had shared that the ancestors of all the rainforest tribes were star people imbued with wisdom and light. Their unified civilization had birthed Evolutionary Science, which included the discipline of sacred plant medicines to help guide humanity through our collective dark night of the soul and back into the natural flow of life. Although I inquired as to the exact time period when Evolutionary Science had originated, Don Sinchi merely grinned at my naivete.

"Such spans of time cannot be measured in years," he said. "My great-grandfather told me that this wisdom comes from time immemorial. It was bequeathed upon our nation by the star beings who, among many other mystical abilities, had tremendous powers to heal others."

As Don Sinchi explained, the two sacred plants, Ayahuasca and Chakruna, were living proof of the Amazonian lineage, representing the complementary opposites of the universe, such as spirit and matter, without which life as we know it would not be possible. The two plants had to be cooked together in order for the medicine of Ayahuasca to be effective. Brought together harmoniously, they awaken the interdimensional nature of our being.

The Path of Heart Mastery: A Blueprint for Awakening

Don Sinchi further shared that the Evolutionary Science of his ancestors contains a blueprint to gradually awaken the higher consciousness from the dream of separation, on both the individual and the collective levels.

The path of Paititi, which is the mastery of the heart's wisdom, branches out into many disciplines. These branches, in the ancient times, encompassed healing, elemental sorcery, raising children, tribal conflict resolution, nourishment of the population, stewarding the health of the rainforest, and many other disciplines. It was clear that the ancients did not see a separation between divine and human matters, as all aspects of human existence were recognized as containing profound meaning on the path of awakening.

In the healing arts branch of Evolutionary Science, for instance, Don Sinchi told me that the ancestors acquired an intimate knowledge of medicinal plants and ways to amplify their healing effects a thousandfold. The enlightened ancestors were also capable of conscious death and rebirth, meaning they could be reborn in a new body while maintaining the memory of their past life, which allowed them to continue their path of service to collective healing, among many other wonders.

"But, Don Sinchi!" I exclaimed impatiently. "If the ancient Amazonians knew all these secrets, how come not all of them were able to survive the fifteenth-century cataclysm?"

The Yahua chief smiled bittersweetly and responded, "They are not secrets but natural expressions of innermost wisdom that each human being has the potential to reach. At the time of the enlightened ancestors, people were intuitively and consistently immersed in unconditional love throughout their everyday existence. When love ruled the world, everyone was free to discover their highest potential, with its accompanying gifts and talents. People would then humbly share their highest potential and encourage each other to do the same."

He went on to explain that, at the time of the cataclysm, only a handful of the Amazonian people were still embodying the evolutionary way of being that enlightened forebears of the lineage cultivated. That was the enlightened stream of awareness, stemming from the original primordial state of Jarichu—the Grandfather Universe who gave birth to complementary opposites, including Father Sun and Mother Earth. It was transmitted to select initiates over thousands of years as a reminder of everyone's true nature.

Once the enlightened ancestors left this dimension of existence, not many of the people left behind were interested in evolutionary reminders. Don Sinchi said, "Most of our people started to lose focus and became satisfied by their narrow specializations in society. In today's world, this same problem is mirrored by people hiding from their issues behind their job titles and egoic accomplishments. The worldwide pandemic of confusion that preceded all physical dis-eases makes us forget the heart's wisdom as the foremost purpose of our existence."

I couldn't help but ask, "Rimyurá, I wonder what made the enlightened ancestors interested in evolutionary reminders?"

Don Sinchi sighed. "In those primordial times, there was nothing but love, which people experienced all the time. It was the most natural and obvious way to be. Because it was so natural, there were no diseases, no wars, and no climate disasters. There were no religions, no traditions, and no spiritual disciplines either, because people were intuitively tuned to the highest, purest frequency of consciousness that abides in the heart's wisdom.

"One day, even before the arrival of the conquistadors, a darkness of unconsciousness descended upon our world. This was the darkness that brought a spiritual amnesia upon the people of the Earth. That was when the wise elders of the time implemented Evolutionary Science. As I've shared, according to our legends, enlightened ancestors lived all across the planet and in continuous communication with each other through their psychic powers. Their ancient precepts formed the human culture that still exists today. The forefathers and foremothers of humanity had also prepared their initiates for the darker times to come."

The chief's face turned serious, and I could detect a tinge of sadness in his voice as he continued: "When the omens of humanity's demise came, brought about by the European outsiders to this region, those initiates who survived the great calamity assembled. Together, they implemented an emergency plan that was prepared in advance for a worst-case scenario."

Don Sinchi explained that, based on indications of ancient prophecies, the originally whole Evolutionary Science was divided into many fragments. Each of these fragments became an ancestral wisdom lineage of its own. This was purposely done as a safety measure since the Evolutionary Science of the ancestors contained too great a power. Originally intended to only be of benefit, in the hands of the ignorant, it could also be used for harm. Ultimately, even plant medicines are instruments that can either cure or poison, depending on who is using them and with what intentions.

Heeding the prophecy to protect this knowledge until humanity will need it most, each tribe became responsible for caretaking distinct facets of ancestral wisdom. Even as fragments, Amazonian lineages carry tremendous power. Initiation rites require a high degree of maturity and accountability that's hard to come across these days. Over the generations, the Amazonian people have only been able to delay, but not prevent, the inevitable dilution of consciousness sweeping the planet.

Don Sinchi elaborated: "Alongside the rest of the world, many of my fellow natives nowadays have forgotten how to honor the primordial wisdom of which they themselves were once an integral element. Instead, they misuse the very heritage that was meant for complete resolution of suffering to indulge in selfish, mystical powers.

"Many ripples of destructive forgetfulness came as a result of consciousness's steady decline, coupled with colonization of this part of the world. It was not in the best interest of the Spaniards to recognize our Indigenous people as civilized. There was a code of honor that existed in Europe at that time regarding encounters with unknown, civilized nations. Instead, it was much more profitable to declare our people savages. The conquistadors were the real savages, however. They pillaged and plundered, driven by primitive greed in this 'new world' of theirs, which, in reality, was our ancient home. They went to great lengths to destroy whatever signs there were of a culture that existed before them. I'm sad to say it, but they were mostly successful.

"Continuous aftershocks of that tragic event have followed since, like the rubber boom, invasion by mining and logging corporations, deforestation, drug trafficking, and the many wars that ignited between the newly erected countries of South America, all the way until now. Our Yahua tribe was lucky enough not to be disturbed until the nineteenth century, when the rubber boom occurred. Then, the wars between Colombia, Chile, Ecuador, Venezuela, Bolivia, and Peru dispersed our people throughout the newly established, illusory borders of this region."

I came to understand that, despite all the waves of destruction, the seed of primordial wisdom still managed to grow—that was how powerful the original tree of Evolutionary Science was. Today, the people of the Amazon—as well as those who are thoroughly committed to the path of heart mastery—are left to caretake the seeds.

Tool: Sowing and Integrating the Seeds of Primordial Wisdom

What are the seeds of your own heart's calling? To nurture the seeds (or to get a sense of what they are if you don't exactly know), reflect on reminders of what makes your heart open more. These may encompass specific activities, practices, subject matters, locations, people, philosophies, etc. Get a sense of how all of it makes you feel in your body (for example, you might feel a sense of spaciousness, ease, flow, vitality, etc.). Do what you can to integrate that which makes your heart open on a daily basis—but even more, train your attention on the embodied states associated with these phenomena, so that you can cultivate them throughout your life.

The Nighthawk's View

As the last of his medicine lineage, Don Sinchi shared with me that his ancestors dealt with so many of the same existential questions that modern people are struggling with today, around issues such as old age, sickness, loss of loved ones, and death. Whereas today our collective generally avoids these matters, the ancestors saw them as rites of passage that bring spiritual maturation and greater meaning into everyday life.

I felt deeply grateful that Don Sinchi was entrusting me with all this information, but he shrugged off my gratitude and said, "To share with you is nothing else but the opportunity for me to fulfill my life's purpose. It doesn't make you special in any way, so don't let it go to your head. Your life circumstances simply humbled you enough to genuinely listen, but if you are not careful, you might lose that ability just as fast!"

The elder continued, "Over the course of my life, I've met some very important Western scientists who came to study our existence. Most of them, however, were convinced that we are crude barbarians. Nothing I could say would've changed their belief systems and perspective about us. So, I told them what they expected to hear: The spirit realm is just like everyday life, abounding with monkeys, parrots, and snakes. None of them ever suspected that I was referring to the monkeying, parroting, and sneakiness of their minds, so indoctrinated with their superiority to Mother Nature."

Don Sinchi looked at me humorously, adding: "At the end of the day, it doesn't matter to me whether you are Yahua, Ashuar, Huitoto, Shipibo, Cocama, Q'ero, or Gringo. What I care about is whether you treasure profound human values with all of your heart. The original name of all tribes in the rainforest is translated into nothing more and nothing less than 'a human being.' The greatest healers of the past here in the Amazon did not identify themselves with any of the tribes and were available to both learn from and share their wisdom with everyone."

Suddenly, Don Sinchi pointed his finger to his ear, signaling for me to be quiet and listen. Initially, I couldn't distinguish any difference from the cacophony of sounds produced by the rainforest around us. Then, I began to hear a piercing whistle, resembling a high-pitched laughter, coming from nearby. He leaned toward me and whispered, "It's a Huancahui nighthawk, out hunting for its favorite food—poisonous snakes. These hawks only come out at night, during the snakes' active hours. We should get going before the ground is covered with wriggling serpents."

I instantly sprang to my feet, and Don Sinchi handed me one of the pails filled with water. He warned me that the snakes were attracted to fear and instructed me to be unafraid, yet fully alert, and to watch my every step. Unable to see much under my feet, I tried to closely follow the steps of the Yahua chief. He was slightly ahead of me, slipping away into impermeable darkness.

We walked quietly through the nighttime rainforest, which reverberated with piercing sounds, before finally reaching Don Sinchi's house. As we put the buckets of water down, I let out a loud sigh of relief. Returning from the creek without the moonlight had taken much longer, and I was glad to find safety from the blood-curdling rainforest, infested with deadly snakes.

The elder swiftly turned toward me, looking intently into my eyes with a piercing, hawklike stare. Noticing my discomfort under his gaze, he said matter-of-factly, "I'd like to share a word of caution with you: You may soon forget all I have just told you.

Poisonous snakes feed on the fear-based mentality that is found in all those who are seeking instant gratification, without any concern for the timeless values of our origins. Instead of avoiding issues, try to view them as rites of passage. Spirit spoke tonight; only with the bird's-eye view of the nighthawk can you become free from the sickness of humanity. Learn to free yourself from the preconceived notions of what is good and bad in your life. Where bad can never become good, the awareness of ignorance is already the seed of wisdom."

Making Love to the Holy Spirit

I was enchanted by the elder's storytelling, which connected me more deeply to my own understanding of what I wanted and why I was here in the first place. Yes, I was in search of a way to move through my life-altering illness, but I wanted something even deeper than a cure. I'd had enough superficial pleasures in my life, and I could see that there was neither real freedom nor lasting happiness in them. Like many Westerners disillusioned by the lure of consumerism and the notion that we can "buy" our way out of the existential struggles that Don Sinchi had discussed with me, I had come to realize that discovering my life's higher purpose was what truly mattered to me. If I could find a way to "remember" myself despite the collective plague of spiritual amnesia, it seemed to me that my struggles could be turned into a meaningful lesson.

The elder smacked his lips thoughtfully and replied, "We'll see how you do in the upcoming Ayahuasca ceremonies, and I will share with you what I know in the meanwhile."

A knot of anticipation had formed in my stomach. I'd been learning a lot from the elder already; his wisdom seemed exhaustive, but as both of us knew, I'd come here seeking out Ayahuasca, because that was what the Amazonian tradition was most known for in the West. I understood that it was an important part of my journey, but I also knew that there was so much more to this Evolutionary Science I was learning. All the same, I was excited to take part in my first Ayahuasca ceremony. I was committed to deepening my studies with Don Sinchi by communing with this powerful medicine.

His smile reminded me of a cat who'd just caught his meal. "Now," he looked around at the rainforest shrouded in the night, "come, and I will show you the *dieta* hut where you'll be staying. In the early morning I must go and gather the medicine to cook. Tomorrow night will be our first ceremony together with you."

As I followed the Yahua chief to my new dwelling, I asked, "Don Sinchi, can I come along with you tomorrow to help collect the medicine?"

The elder frowned. "Absolutely not. Much purification is needed before you can ask permission from the rainforest spirit to collect the sacred plants. Without proper preparation, a poisonous snake will bite you, for sure. Just rest for now. Tomorrow, we will be dieting on farinha and grilled plantains all day long. The diet of bland physical food helps reveal the subtle taste of our innermost purpose as the source and nourishment of all that exists in the universe. Such discipline trains our body, mind, and spirit to connect with our true selves without distractions."

Seeing my disappointed smile, he added: "This dieta has many more reasons behind it; however, the main one for you right now is to let go of the earthly pleasures that usually dominate life and reconnect to the subtle senses of your higher self. I hope you have not had pork, alcohol, or sex for the past three days, for your own sake."

I was familiar with spiritual traditions that promote abstinence, but I wondered aloud as to why it was so important preceding an Ayahuasca ceremony.

Don Sinchi replied, "A medicine woman friend of mine refers to the ceremony of Ayahuasca as making love to the Holy Spirit. Ayahuasca is a goddess of Mother Nature, and a very jealous one at that. She can see as well as a nighthawk whether we value the most profound and unconditional expression of love or prefer the cheap substitutes of instant gratifications."

The elder explained that it takes time to cultivate a loving relationship with the Ayahuasca plant spirit. The dieta helps bring deeper and clearer intentions into one's life. To be worthy of merely glimpsing the goddess, we must prepare ourselves by interrupting the vicious cycle of futile attempts to fill the void, which often entails earthly pleasures that give us a sense of passing comfort that can prevent our growth. Most importantly, we need the dieta to release our cravings and lift our consciousness into Mother Nature's life force. In other words, the dieta helps transmute the lower vibrations into the more sublime qualities necessary for our evolution.

I suddenly heard what I thought was a snake slithering through the leaves nearby. I jolted my head in the direction of the sound, just in time to see a leaf the size of a beach umbrella landing on the ground outside my hut. When I turned my head back to Don Sinchi, he was nowhere in sight. The Yahua elder had mysteriously vanished into the night, without making a sound.

After such an eventful day, I was happy to get some rest. Lying in the cocoon of my mosquito net that night, I felt like a fetus in Mother Nature's womb. My reasoning mind was subdued by the mesmerizing stories I'd heard. Although I'd just met Don Sinchi, it felt like I'd known him forever.

Tool: Evolving with the Help of a Dieta

As Don Sinchi shared with me, the dieta offers ways to connect with the true self, free of distractions or comforts that may keep you stuck in a state of spiritual stasis, unable to evolve into who you are meant to be. Beyond food restrictions, a dieta can involve changing the habitual patterns in your life so that instead of attempting to "fill the void," you can begin to honor what is truly meaningful for you. Reflect and journal on more fulfilling and meaningful ways you can engage your time. Create a dieta that is free of instant gratifications and filled with ways to nurture greater meaning that lasts a few days, one day, or even just a few hours to start.

REFLECTIONS

- Interconnectedness and reciprocity are universal laws that define the foundation of our individual and shared existence. Our intentions create this realm of appearances, just as imagination creates images out of the mist. Because of ignorance, the original heaven on Earth has gotten lost in the smoke-and-mirror aberrations of the human mind. *In what ways do you tangibly experience interconnectedness and reciprocity in your own life? In what ways do you struggle with experiencing these universal laws in a direct way?*

- Don Sinchi shared that in the very beginning of human civilizations, people didn't have specific spiritual paths, because they naturally abided in a state of unconditional love. The lineages were created as reminders to return to that original heart-centered state. *What are the lineages, spiritual traditions, and cultures in your life that help you remember to come back into the heart?*

- To see clearly, with the view of the nighthawk, you must be willing to relinquish your fear of the shadows lurking in the unconscious mind. *In what ways are you ruled by fear? In what ways might you be able to let it go, to be ushered into the light of clear wisdom?*

- Mother Nature is constantly offering us extraordinary ways to commune with her wisdom, and thus, be reconnected to our own nature. Don Sinchi shared that the enlightened ancestors of the Amazon rainforest offered Ayahuasca and Chakruna as sacred plants that would help reconnect humans with the essence of primordial wisdom. *In what ways has nature been a teacher to you?*

CHAPTER 3

THE FIRST
CEREMONY

The time for the first Ayahuasca ceremony had come after the sun set the next day.

I observed Don Sinchi smoking a local tobacco variety from his pipe. This was *mapacho*, which he later informed me was another sacred plant in the rainforest that channeled the intentions of the healer and also purified negative energy. He leaned over a ceramic vessel with geometric designs painted on it and unplugged the wooden cork at the top of the container, which was filled to the brim with a dark brown liquid. After a moment of silence, Don Sinchi started whistling a tune while blowing the mapacho smoke, infused with his healing energy, into the Ayahuasca brew. It was clear to me that I was in the presence of a holy rite.

While Don Sinchi was praying, more people timidly walked inside the *maloka* (the hut where the ceremony would be held) one by one. Some of them appeared to be Yahua, and some were mestizo. Each person silently bowed to the elder before finding a place for themselves against the wall. Once everyone had gathered, Don Sinchi finished his invocations over the medicine and gently set the ceramic vessel aside.

Standing up, the elder began addressing everyone in the room: "All of us gathered here in the womb of the maloka are about to enter a sacred ceremony with the medicine of our ancestors. This medicine is renowned for her ability to heal many issues plaguing humankind, including physical diseases, since time immemorial."

Don Sinchi explained that Ayahuasca is not always pleasant or comfortable, because she allows us to face and heal all that we usually sweep under the carpet of our own ignorance. Repressed emotions, fears, and inhibitions can all come up to the surface, but they are always there in service of our transformation.

He continued, "The ceremony involves purging whatever toxins have accumulated in your being throughout this lifetime and beyond. Whether physical, emotional, or mental, it all must be expelled with the grace of Mother Nature. Remember that you are not getting sick during the ceremony, but are releasing all that is not natural to your being. Be grateful for that.

"The ceremony is guided with the divine *icaros* that were passed down through the ages. These are melodies from the time when our ancestors were in profound communion with Mother Nature. These icaros will illuminate the pathways for you to navigate the ocean of the Great Spirit."

He went on to explain that, in the beginning of the ceremony, he would invoke a magical circle of protection around the maloka, so that any negative energies would be expelled from the circle without the possibility of reentry. Especially for those of us, like myself, who were just beginning to know this medicine, it was essential to remain within the circle as much as possible. It was permissible to walk outside to the bathroom, or to purge, or to get some fresh air when needed, but we were asked to return as quickly as we could to the sacred circle—or we might fall prey to the negative energies that had been asked to leave.

The Yahua elder paused, lit his pipe, and blew smoke in the different directions of the maloka. He kept silent for a while, sitting with his eyes closed, and then started whistling quietly, occasionally puffing smoke.

I sat there, anxiously waiting for us to start, but he did not seem to be in a hurry. He was completely at ease and without a worry in the world. It occurred to me that Don Sinchi was counterbalancing the palpable trepidation coming from me and the others gathered together that night. Just acknowledging the contrast between his state and the rest of us helped me snap out of the fear that had started to overtake me just moments before.

It was time to remember who I really was.

A Lesson from a Tree

The elder, as if responding to the harmonization of energy in the room, spoke again: "Although I will be here for you throughout the whole ceremony, it's essential for you to learn how to face your own challenges. That's how the strength of your spirit evolves: by discovering that you are capable of a lot more than you think. However, in case you are struggling to the point of despair, know that you can always call upon me to guide you through your experience.

"During the challenging moments, it's crucial to invoke all that is sacred in your life, not only for yourself, but for all the beings who suffer and are lost in the darkness of their ignorance. We learn during these ceremonies to face the adversities of everyday life with a deep, peaceful presence by trusting in the Great Spirit to provide us with exactly what is needed to continue our evolutionary journey as children of the universe."

Don Sinchi stopped talking and met each of the people in the room with a stern yet kind gaze. There were 13 of us in the maloka; as we took our turns receiving the medicine, he blessed us individually, offering the cup while we approached him in the dim candlelight.

When my turn came, I slowly walked over to the Rimyurá. I realized that Don Sinchi was seeing right through me with his piercing hawk eyes. He nodded after a moment. He then carefully measured the sacrament into a decorated cup made from the hard shell of the huito fruit. He whistled an incantation into the cup and handed it to me. I took a whiff of the liquid inside; the smell was nauseatingly sweet. Deciding not to prolong the potentially terrible taste, I took a quick shot of the thick, brown liquid, emptying the cup all at once. The sacrament had a strangely familiar taste I could not quite place, but it wasn't as bad as I'd imagined it might be. Proud of myself for not recoiling from the aftertaste, like some of the other people who had taken the potion before me, I returned to my seat.

After about a half hour of not feeling any effects whatsoever, I started wondering whether I was immune to the medicine. But suddenly, I felt inebriated, and strangely, simultaneously sober. Vibrations reverberated throughout my being until thoughts, sensations, and images began merging as one. Pulsating colors bubbled up from my belly, rising to my throat. I barely had enough time to get outside before a strong purge erupted from me.

After a while, I returned to the maloka. I felt sick and exhausted from all the purging. I was silently swearing to myself many times over that I would never, *ever*, do anything like this again. Thinking about how I didn't want to continue with the experience was only making it worse. At times, I felt intense pain in places where my body was already sick. Then, the physical pain would transform and be replaced by disturbing emotions. After some time, emotional and mental anguish morphed into visuals of deformed creatures and distorted, agonized-looking faces.

I sat in a state of stupefaction as I realized that Ayahuasca was showing me how my unconscious resistance to various situations in my life had caused my body to become sick. For example, I would often feel very uncomfortable and awkward in social situations because I felt unable to pretend everything was fine in my life—business as usual. My stomach would tense in an instinctive reaction to a world in which vulnerability was not welcomed. Because of this continuous tension, the flow of oxygen and blood circulation to my digestive tract was greatly diminished, contributing to my inability to heal myself. The natural flow of life force, distorted by my conditioning, was affecting my physical state, as well as my emotional, sensory, and mental faculties. This had been the cause of so much suffering in my life.

I ran outside again to purge. Upon finally being done, amazing lightness and clarity filled my being. The sickness and exhaustion I'd felt just moments before was completely gone! I was suddenly able to tune in to the icaros and prayers. Don Sinchi's melodies fell like a rain of blessings from the heavens, imbuing my entire being with Universal Love and resonance with all of creation. I hadn't even acknowledged his presence until that point in the ceremony, being so wrapped up in my misery.

Although that wonderful state continued to be interspersed with physical and emotional purges, I could handle the process much better from that point on, since I'd already been shown the potential of peace and serenity by the spirit of the medicine.

Don Sinchi invited me to come and sit in front of him for a *limpia* (a cleansing and healing ritual). As I approached him, he whispered to me, "Do you hear the music of Mother Nature?"

I listened attentively to the variety of sounds that the rainforest was producing in awesome unison all around the maloka. The song of the rainforest was traveling in shimmering waves through my awareness.

"Yes, I hear her."

Don Sinchi continued to speak with a soft and clear voice: "That is her way of expressing unconditional love to the infinite mystery surrounding us."

The Rimyurá then began whistling the most magnificently haunting melody, which wasn't just heard by my ears, but rhythmically pulsated through every particle of my being. I simultaneously saw and felt a kaleidoscopic snake (a common motif in Ayahuasca ceremonies) moving inside me, liberating energetic blockages within my being. As the limpia came to completion, the elder blew mapacho smoke into my hands and over the top of my head. Immediately, the sensory overload swept over me again and I frantically ran outside to purge a stream of rainbow spiders. Feeling even more cleansed, yet thoroughly exhausted by this particular purge, I returned to the maloka and lay in a fetal position on the earthen floor.

Although I felt much better physically, I was still troubled by the same nagging question that had brought me to the Amazon in the first place. It had to do with what Don Sinchi had asked the night before: "What is the purpose of your life?"

No matter how hard I tried, I could not find an answer. After yet another epic purge outside the maloka, I experienced deep sadness and desperation while reflecting on my life's meaning. Noticing my mind drifting off, I returned my focus to my breath. Suddenly, I found myself interwoven with a myriad of rainforest sounds. My body, responding to nature's soundscape, also began dancing along with the aliveness mirrored to me from all directions.

Through the symphony of countless life-forms, an idea came to me that I should ask a tree about *its* life purpose. Perhaps it would bring me closer to understanding my own purpose. Despite my rational mind's resistance to such a ridiculous notion, I looked around and saw a tree that seemed approachable. I carefully stepped toward it with my now-uncoordinated body, which, with the influence of the Ayahuasca, was dancing sporadically of its own accord. Then, I asked the existential question that had been troubling me so much.

Surprisingly, the tree responded telepathically, with a loud voice inside my head: "I can't answer this question for you, but that other tree can."

Somehow, the tree pointed me to another tree a short distance away. Immediately, I discerned that there was something very different about this tree. It was a tall, old, majestic tree with a beam of bright, white light extending from its crown toward the sky. I went over to the magnificent tree and placed my hand on its trunk. As soon as I did, it ceased to be a tree. Instead, it transformed into an immense, oval-shaped energy field, bursting with luminosity.

"Tree, what is your purpose?" I asked.

As soon as I asked that question, something inexplicable happened. I almost recoiled in shock as a powerful energy surged through the luminous field of the tree and into the very core of my being. With it, I heard the tree's answer: "*This* is what I live for!"

The energy of the tree grew brighter and brighter as innumerable ripples of light were discharged into my body. The tree kept repeating itself, with each new wave of light sweeping over me: "This is what I live for—I live for *this*!"

Each time, the ripples of light became more and more dazzling, until there was nothing but brilliant, peaceful light everywhere— and I was inseparable from it.

Tool: What Do You Live For?

Take some time to contemplate and journal: What are the inspirations, passions, and hobbies that engage your innermost spark? Reflect on how you can unite all of them under the greater umbrella of a higher purpose in your life. A multidisciplinary approach to life, which the ancestors embodied, when translated into our modern context, will look different for everyone. For example, if you are a medical doctor, your passion for painting can help bring greater precision to your healing arts in an operating room. Be creative and expansive as you consider the ways in which your gifts might coalesce to bring meaning into your life and power into your contributions.

Awakening Spiritual Sight

Once I was back in the healing circle of the maloka, I continued to experience the waves and undercurrents of eternal life force cradling me. The icaros felt like they were planting brilliant seeds in my wide-open heart throughout the rest of the night. Only toward the early morning did our ceremony come to its completion, and the medicine gradually receded into the mystery of Nature within each of us.

After most of the participants had left, Don Sinchi walked over and looked at me with curiosity and a kind smile. He told me to head back to my hut and rest so that the healing could continue on subtler levels.

I woke up after about four hours to the song of forest birds. Even though my stomach had been through hell during the ceremony, I felt like my entire being had been reborn. I was physically tired from the intensity of last night's healing, but my mind was very much lucid and aware.

Outside, I saw Don Sinchi's daughter, Warmi, approaching my hut, carrying something in her hands. She saw that I was awake, so she came in and greeted me cheerfully. She handed me a cup she was carrying—it was lemon juice with crushed garlic mixed with water. She shared that her father recommended it to everyone after the ceremonies to regenerate the liver and rejuvenate the body after all the detoxing.

She was right; as I drank, I immediately felt refreshed and soothed.

On her way out, she said, "My father asked to see you once you get up—you will find him in the maloka."

I took a moment to enjoy the harmonious hum of nature. As I walked toward the maloka, I listened to the chirping of the birds and couldn't help but feel a sense of renewal of hope for myself and the rest of our modern world.

Once I was back inside the maloka, I found Don Sinchi in the same spot he'd been sitting in during the ceremony, as if he'd never left. In the daylight, I could see that the maloka was a round wooden house, with an earthen floor covered in white sand and windows that were completely shut during the ceremonies to prevent even the tiniest ray of light from seeping through. The ceremonial temple was shorn of decorations. The barren appearance surprised me, as I knew how sacred this place was for the Indigenous people.

"You must wonder why there are no pictures in my temple," Don Sinchi said after greeting me and reading my thoughts, as he always seemed to. "Some medicine men and women today have skulls, exotic ornaments, and flashy garments. Others have exquisite altars and even dead condors hanging in their temples, while I only have this."

He smiled while pointing to the center of his forehead. "Which comes from here." Then, he pointed to the center of his chest. "You see, Romancito, in the ceremony, our mind turns on like a light bulb, and reality transforms. When you learn to focus your inner eye, you will see us transported into a crystal palace with a mesmerizing altar appearing before me. You can also see all the people in the ceremony, based on the vibration of their consciousness. That kind of seeing is very different from how you perceive reality through your physical eyes."

"Is that why the ceremonies take place in pitch-black darkness, Don Sinchi?" I asked.

"Yes, the darkness helps awaken our spiritual sight. During the ceremony, this maloka becomes a cosmic womb for the light-seed of the Great Spirit to sprout in your heart, helping you become a light unto yourself."

He then asked how my night had been. I related my experiences, no matter how incoherent they had been—except for the tree encounter, which I'd encountered in perfect lucidity.

Don Sinchi asked me to show him the special tree I'd conversed with. When I brought him to it, his face lit up.

"This is a White Lupuna tree—she is the greatest teacher of wisdom among all the trees of the rainforest. This particular Lupuna is the youngest one in the area, at about 130 years of age. My great-grandfather planted it long before my parents were born. I see it as a very good sign that Ayahuasca brought you to her."

Illness as Initiation

After we headed back to the maloka, Don Sinchi shared, "I saw you last night in my visions. You certainly did not come here by chance, because you have a mark that drives you, tree talker! How is the problem in your intestines?"

I was stunned for a good moment. I had never told him or anyone else; he knew about the Crohn's disease I'd had since the age of 12, which was one of my main motivations for coming to the Amazon in the first place.

My thoughts raced as I looked for some logical explanation for the fact that he knew something I'd never disclosed. After a long pause, I finally managed to squeeze a few words out. "Yes, I have this . . . mark, but how did you know that?"

Don Sinchi pointed to the ceramic vessel he'd poured the sacrament from last night, reminding me, "As I already told you, with the help of this medicine, people's true colors come out in the ceremony—and that is what allows the transformation to occur. Accepting what the Great Spirit reveals allows us to come to terms with ourselves. Only then can all our troubles be healed."

I was a little puzzled with what he was saying, so I responded, "My Western upbringing taught me to resist what bothers me, not to accept it. That seems to be contrary to what you are saying, Don Sinchi."

The elder smiled and quickly became serious once again. After a prolonged silence, he explained, "The world of society and the realm of the Great Spirit are very different domains, and in each there are specific rules and guidelines of being. In our modern world, people are raised to become useful members of society. The current civilization is not interested in our development as human beings. Instead of exploring this essential subject, people are taught narrow specializations, with very little connection to the wholehearted wish of benefiting the greater whole. People are conditioned to be mindlessly domesticated puppets of the mainstream system; they are driven by external rewards like power over others, fleeting pleasures, and financial status. That kind of indoctrination reduces consciousness to a herd mentality. Driven by external recognition and rewards, people lose inner peace and try to get the best for themselves, while avoiding the worst at all costs."

"Well, that makes sense," I told Don Sinchi. "In my world, that's exactly how things work."

"Of course it makes sense—you are a product of that system! What is best and what is worst was already decided for you before you were born. People today grow into specific molds of expectations, successes, failures, and regrets that shape them into who they are. As a human race, we continue to instill the same programming into all the new generations. Each member of society who is unaware of this vicious cycle keeps reinforcing it in everyone around them. The mystery of being then gets lost in superficial values, like a pearl in mud!

"In the modern world, people are taught everything except the most essential thing: how to live life to the fullest! In the world of Mother Nature, on the other hand, that is the main focus—and things obviously work quite differently because of that. Without acknowledging the basic predicament of being alive here on Earth for only a short time, people lose themselves in superficial values. Consequently, without true care for each other, our highest potential will never fully awaken. What if I tell you, for example, that your disease is a blessing and not a curse? You might not see it now, but in due time, all in due time . . . "

I sighed to myself. I couldn't imagine how I might begin seeing my illness in a positive light.

Don Sinchi continued, "In our tradition, both the healer and the patient have equal responsibility in the evolutionary healing journey; the healer must make sure that the patient is not seeing them as a messiah, but as a friend who means well and knows what that means. No one, not even an enlightened ancestor, can do the work for you. The teacher provides the clear direction from a more objective perspective, and the student must verify the guidance they received via a direct personal initiative. 'Trust, but check' is the foundational principle of our lineage."

Don Sinchi then asked me to share the details of my illness with him. Still very lucid and receptive after last night's ceremony, I noticed right away that my body contracted in response to his request. I realized how, over the course of my life, I had developed a fear of vulnerability. Being in the maloka suddenly took me back into the healing experience from the previous night. My awareness was flooded with the realizations I'd had under the effects of the medicine. What I'd glimpsed in my first ceremony with the Yahua elder was the willingness to face myself and my predicaments fully. Right away, the spark of my spirit became brighter than the need to judge my suffering. The fear of sharing my unresolved issues dissolved.

"The healing journey began for me at the age of twelve with a medical diagnosis of Crohn's disease in my colon. The illness is genetic, incurable, and ultimately terminal, according to Western allopathic medicine. My gastroenterologist once shared with me that, in terms of its location in the body and the pain during the acute phases, it's the closest experience a man could have to giving birth.

"Approximately five years after being diagnosed, my prescribed conventional pharmaceuticals stopped helping me, making me feel much worse instead. After a series of additional tests, the doctors confirmed that my body no longer responded favorably to their medication. I was informed that if the condition continued to deteriorate, my only option would be to operate. Conventional treatment involved surgically removing the portions of my large intestine that were most affected by the condition. Because the source of the disease itself was not being treated, the deterioration would only progress with time. Therefore, invasive surgeries would have to continue for the rest of my life. In fact, my paternal grandmother, from whom I inherited the condition, had multiple surgeries throughout the last forty years of her life. She passed away from complications after her last surgery. So, as you might understand, these solutions weren't appealing to me at all. I suddenly became motivated to search for alternative healing options far and wide. Eventually, my search led me here, to the Amazon."

Don Sinchi listened attentively and finally exclaimed, "Don't you see now how this illness brought you to the path of your heart? It sounds like a part of you wished for the illness to happen! And what your gastroenterologist told you about childbirth pain is in line with our people's ancestral view of dis-eases as reminders of being born. You have been gestating in the womb of your dis-ease long enough to start evolving beyond your fetal state! All that has happened and continues to happen in your life is meant to help you finally birth your true self into existence."

Observing my bewildered reaction to what he was saying, Don Sinchi elaborated: "Everything in the environment of the ancients was natural, including the sicknesses, which were honored as messengers of the Great Spirit. The diseases were referred to as 'merciless mothers.' As a healer, I continue to honor these ancestral ways. The diseases are recognized in our tradition as wake-up calls from the collective dream of separation and rites of passage into one's higher purpose. The return to the Mother's womb, through illness, is about remembering essential human qualities and what it means to be whole again. Without remembrance, it's not possible to become a real human being in a body and subsequently heal."

"Wouldn't I be more whole without my sickness?" I asked, slightly confused.

"You would, but first you have to live through it and be born from it! Once the essential human qualities are remembered, you can return to society, reborn in your higher purpose, to begin life anew. The world then becomes a training ground for those awe-inspiring qualities that can transform all your habits of resistance into creative life.

"Our people's view of healing is quite radical, considering the modern, conventional medicine approach. In your world, people submit to the mercy of the medical establishment, just to keep their 'normal' routines."

He started to imitate fainting while moaning, "Please put me to sleep and do whatever you want for all my problems to go away! My life is everyone else's fault, and I am not responsible for it!"

Suddenly, he rubbed his eyes with both hands, like someone who'd just awakened out of delirium.

"You see, Romancito, people in the modern world are conditioned to see disease as something that prevents them from living their 'normal' lives. It's convenient to see illnesses as bothersome and random, lacking any meaning or higher purpose. The real disease, of course, is the pandemic of forgetfulness. Spiritual amnesia is the main contributing factor to modern society's obsession with the consumerist existence.

"In the perspective of modern medicine, the symptoms of the disease must be destroyed, surgically removed, burned, or poisoned, even at the cost of killing the patient, as in the case of chemotherapy and radiation treatments. Yet, without considering its lifestyle, values, and belief systems as the main culprits, modern society chooses the quantity of meaningless years on this Earth over the quality of life experience, which goes on beyond this temporary existence. If we don't consciously engage ignorance as the root of suffering, it'll keep making itself known, through a great multitude of symptoms."

I asked Don Sinchi to elaborate further on the differences he saw between the modern medical approach and his ancestral healing tradition. He thought about it for a moment and then got up, replying, "Come join me on a walk to my medicinal plant nursery, and you might hear something useful along the way."

Tool: Facing and Birthing Your
True Self into Existence

Reflect on the dis-ease in your life. This may not necessarily be a physical affliction. What bothers you? What feels disempowering and unfulfilling? View all that as the dark womb of your conditioning.

Now, look at all the inspirations in your life as the complementary opposites of all the disappointment that has gestated in your heart. Even being stuck in a meaningless nine-to-five job can help you develop an immense motivation to actualize your talents and develop a strategy of following your heart. Contemplate which activities in your life can bring about the positive qualities that are waiting to be born into practical application on a steady basis. Include these activities in your own personal dieta.

REFLECTIONS

- Each of us and all life-forms are the connecting links between Mother Earth and the vast universe. As I learned from Don Sinchi, this is what we've come here to realize. When we express the essence of who each of us is, the sacred circle of life heals us, and our awareness of this miraculous existence is continually rekindled. *As you reflect on your own journey, how can you begin to perceive the many ways in which you've been guided here by the call of the Great Spirit? How can you allow that call to help you step even more decisively into your essence so that you can experience it in a more powerful way?*

- The message I received from the elder-tree teacher reverberated through every cell in my body: "Be light and share that light with the world! The more you share your love, the more luminous you'll become." *In what ways do you hold back from sharing your own light with the world? How can you be bolder in choosing to become a light unto yourself?*

- During my first Ayahuasca ceremony, I gradually returned to my body from the blissful realm of all-encompassing luminosity. Despite all the purges, I felt totally refreshed and revitalized, as a newfound realization about my true nature permeated my heart. *What have been some of your own moments of embracing all-encompassing luminosity? How might dipping into these memories help anchor you on your spiritual journey?*

- What we resist persists, but in our Western world, we are taught to view "unfortunate" or "uncomfortable" experiences as things to avoid or escape, rather than opportunities to birth ourselves anew, into our true nature. *What are your chosen methods of avoidance and escape? If you were to shift your perspective so that you could recognize painful opportunities as powerful rites of passage, how would this transmute your experience of difficulty or discomfort?*

CHAPTER 4

IN THE NURSERY OF THE GREAT SPIRIT

What is health and healing? I contemplated this question as Don Sinchi and I left the maloka and began to stroll along one of the many trails leading into the forest.

After some time, Don Sinchi spoke again, in response to where we'd left off: "It's not even 'health' per se, but a lack of symptoms that today's society is after. However, that would mean complete numbness and death. In this life, we cannot avoid pain. It's natural, and our bodies are wired to feel it. Why? Because it's part of our communication system with the higher intelligence of Nature that keeps us engaged in our life's journey."

He went on to explain that most people in today's world are conditioned to see disease as something that prevents them from living their "normal" lives. But in Don Sinchi's Indigenous healing tradition, pain encourages greater love to come through, while diseases are evolutionary catalysts. I was surprised by this paradigm shift from the modern world's conventional view of disease.

He casually continued, smiling at my dumbstruck expression, "On the path of remembering the self as an integral part of the greater whole, an individual is seen as healthy only once they stop dragging their old habits into their new life. That is one of the most essential teachings behind the Ayahuasca tradition. The name itself implies that: *Aya* signifies 'the realm of the dead or realm of

Spirit' and *huasca* means 'a rope or umbilical cord.' The real medicine is the death of the limited, superficial identity and rebirth of Nature, which can never die."

The elder stopped at a turn on the forest trail, cautiously looked around, and then glanced at me. He smiled, noticing my stupefied expression. "Here in the rainforest exists a snakelike, mythical creature that has a head on each side. It's called Sacha-Mama, which translates from the intertribal dialect as 'the Forest Mother.' When you cut one head, another grows in its place. She is indestructible, and the only way to avoid being devoured by her is to pierce her heart with an unwavering, loving presence. This gigantic two-headed serpent symbolizes the uncontainable force of nature within each of us; running away from, fighting, or clinging to forces of nature will only result in self-inflicted harm. Yet, by consciously channeling this uncontainable energy through the heart, we transform the fierce power of nature into healing potential, in service of the greater good."

As the elder took a pause, orienting himself at another fork in the trail, I thought of a parallel metaphor to the Sacha-Mama legend in the West: the so-called double-edged sword, which relates to an experience that has both positive and negative effects. I had never tried to relate with my affliction in such an unconventional way. I found the double-headed snake to be a much better symbol for my dis-ease than an inanimate sword.

Don Sinchi spoke again after a prolonged silence: "Our people's earth-based spirituality values a practical approach. Since dis-ease is inevitable in life, it's much more meaningful to see it as Nature's benevolent intelligence that encourages us to discover our innate healing potential."

Just then, we reached the medicinal plant nursery of the Yahua chief. It consisted of many old decomposing tree trunks laid flat on the ground. The trunks were hollowed out in the shapes of canoes and filled with dark soil. Many plant varieties grew here, under the shade of a thick canopy, created by the interwoven Ayahuasca vines that flourished above. Don Sinchi explained that he kept his medicinal plants nearby because they were his living library and a pharmacy of Mother Nature.

Carefully, so as not to damage the branches growing over the entrance, we entered the nursery. It was Don Sinchi's custom to plant seeds and transplant little saplings after ceremonies, when the connection with Nature is the strongest.

He lovingly began digging his hands into the dark, rich soil to soften it for planting. "As a curandero, I will never go against the disease, because that would mean going against Mother Nature herself. Instead, I go alongside it, listening intently to what the sickness is trying to communicate through each patient. I can then do some inner landscaping and fertilize the soil of people's life experience for the Great Spirit's seeds to be delivered and planted firmly. The messages of the Great Spirit are always communicated on the level of essential human qualities that the patient is deficient in, such as forbearance, patience, self-acceptance, tenderness, and ingenuity, among others. Only once the inner ground is ready for evolutionary remediation can I provide the spiritual first aid for the seeds of humanity within the patient to sprout."

This struck a nerve. I retorted, "I don't see how a mental understanding of the Great Spirit's messages can help me heal from my condition. Also, what do you mean by 'inner soil fertilization' and 'spiritual first aid'?" I felt frustrated by both of Don Sinchi's metaphors and my own inability to decipher them.

Don Sinchi leaned to the side and lifted a small ceramic pot that hid in the thick brush on one side of the nursery. Placing it in front of him, he pulled out a folded leaf filled with rounded seeds. As the elder began patiently planting the seeds, he smiled and replied in a calm, soothing voice: "Preparing the soil is about providing the supportive conditions for the beginner's mind to be born. The spiritual first aid then follows, because it guides and directs these Lupuna seeds to sprout from the dark womb of the Earth toward the light. The seeds of the Great Spirit sprout because an umbilical cord, rooted in the womb of Creation, provides them with vital nourishment.

"What gets us through the darkness of unconscious existence is our search for a higher purpose. Once born into the brilliant awareness of one's infinite potential, the initiate must keep drawing motivation from life's adversities. The challenges in our lives are essential for our potential of fearless love to be fully realized as the Great Spirit. The fertile soil of Pacha Mama, the great Mother Earth, will remain dormant without the seeds of Spirit's light that impregnate Her, as well as all the storms of life that create the perfect conditions for sprouting."

I didn't fully understand what he meant, but his poetic language reminded me of a quote from the Vietnamese Buddhist teacher Thích Nhất Hạnh, "No mud, no lotus," which suggests that openness to adversity liberates us from suffering. The elder proceeded to lovingly cover the Lupuna seeds he'd planted and to pat the earth with his open palms. He got up and observed me intently before lighting his pipe and blowing smoke all over the nursery. We then returned to the maloka through the intricate weaving of rainforest pathways that only Don Sinchi knew how to navigate.

Once we were back inside the maloka, Don Sinchi invited me to sit next to him. He closed his eyes; after contemplatively puffing on his pipe for a few minutes, he finally spoke: "What I shared with you today was to demonstrate that conceptual understanding can only encourage the cultivation of wisdom but cannot replace it.

"The wisdom I am speaking of is the Motherly Wisdom, earned through unwavering dedication to keeping the heart open, no matter the circumstances. Conceptual logic can never substitute Nature's wisdom, which births all life into the world.

"The embodiment of Nature's wisdom, however, depends solely on your discipline applied to your healing journey. There's a Spanish saying, *A mal tiempo buena cara*, which basically means, 'Keep a good attitude in troubled times.' That is the foundation of inner discipline in our tradition."

The Ancestral Diagnosis of Dis-ease

I wanted to understand how I could acquire this wisdom that Don Sinchi spoke so humbly yet so passionately about. On some level, I understood that it was my own ignorance and resistance that continued to block me. I wanted rational explanations for these blockages, but from everything Don Sinchi was sharing, they wouldn't take me too far.

"Don Sinchi, I understand that dis-ease provides a way for us to come back to Nature's wisdom. But I want to know why we get sick. How do these blockages that lead to dis-ease occur in the first place?"

He replied, "In our Amazonian healing tradition, we have our own diagnostic system of various conditions that block aliveness in the organism. They are shared across all tribes with corresponding terms that are commonly referenced nowadays among most Amazonian healers, native and mestizo alike."

He explained that there are five main pathologies the Amazonian healing system deals with:

1. *Saladera is related to stagnation caused by the consumerist mentality of trying to fill the void with junk food and other disempowering coping mechanisms. It's often accompanied by a sense of bad luck and self-deprecation.*

2. *Susto is a paralyzing trauma from a fearful shock that most often occurs in childhood but can also affect people throughout most of their adult lives. It can affect the metabolism, as well as the nervous and immune systems.*

3. *Pulsario has to do with the lack of willpower and depletion of vital force due to unresolved emotional knots. It's accompanied by self-pity, deficiency of nutrients, and depletion of vitality.*

4. *Mal ojo is based on a lack of connection to others that causes envy to ensue. It's accompanied by an absence of inner peace, consequently making people lose weight from stress and insomnia.*

5. *Daño is a more progressive version of mal ojo, and it occurs when people intentionally seek revenge, blaming their unresolved issues on others. This condition can lead to liver and heart problems, as well as the sense of a dark cloud hovering over the self, causing all kinds of inner and outer misfortunes.*

"These are some examples of how ignorance causes suffering," he said before pausing to puff smoke in the different directions of the maloka, as he chanted an incantation in the Yahua language. I understood based on his intonation and body language that he was expelling the negative energies that had been left over after the ceremony. I inquired as to why this was necessary.

He gave me his impersonal signature smile. "By sharing with you how the poison of ignorance causes suffering, I have tapped into these distorted energies in myself and also everyone with whom I'm energetically connected through the ceremonial work. The healing circle of the ceremony is the womb of Mother Nature's unconditional love. All the people from last night's ceremony are still connected to me through the natural state of being bestowed upon them by the Ayahuasca spirit. I am sending all of them continuous healing intentions through the mapacho smoke to help them illuminate their ignorance. If I don't do that and close my heart to patients as soon as I close the ceremony, then I am no better than a sideshow attraction. Their ignorance will then amplify mine, dimming the light of nature within and creating a swampy darkness of heavy vibrations in this maloka instead.

"While it's possible for me to temporarily dissipate the clouds of ignorance during the ceremony so that people can get a glimpse of their true nature, the real healing must come through each individual's own motivation in every moment of life. The conditions I described to you just now are direct consequences of specific poisons that form from the absence of emotional intelligence. These unconscious tendencies steal people's souls, which is another way to say that people lose their wholeness."

He went on to explain that fear of the unknown, which relates to confusion, is what causes *pulsario* and *susto*. Craving results in *saladera* and bad luck. Envy causes *mal ojo*; even if someone else gave it to you, they are still a mirror of the way you inwardly treat yourself. Aggression, when either suppressed within or constantly reacted upon outwardly, attracts *daño*.

He noted that in each case, a distinct soul retrieval process (which allows a person to return to a natural state of wholeness) that's relevant to the person's individual predicament is required.

Once the soul is retrieved, it's up to the individual to keep their soul alive and vibrant in every moment. The first step is to stop perpetuating the specific expression of ignorance that caused the problem in the first place. When virtuous qualities are simultaneously cultivated alongside a reversal of the individual's conditioning, these qualities become a balm for the soul. The soul's innocence, which was wounded, begins to heal.

I said, "This is an interesting theory, but how is it practically applied?"

He looked at me and replied, "Well, for one, you can stop being angry at yourself for being angry. The only way to retrieve the soul and keep our spirits high through all the hardships of life is to remedy the poisons of our ignorance with essential human qualities. Of course, ceremonies can help us get a strong glimpse of our innate wholeness. However, our innate primordial essence is supported by the continuous cultivation of such qualities as openness, sincerity, kindness, compassion, patience, generosity, perseverance, and many others that reflect the organic intelligence of Mother Nature that I already mentioned.

"We are all created in the image of Nature's unconditional love and are familiar with her wisdom since before our birth. Your inner yearning to reunite with the heart of all the hearts is the umbilical cord between Mother Nature and all her creations. It can never be severed. However, it's up to each of us to consciously receive her boundless Wisdom of the Heart. The essential human qualities together comprise the umbilical cord that connects each of us to our highest purpose. By honoring these qualities, you nurture the seeds of the heart's potential. Once born into the light of your life's deepest meaning, you must continue to embrace the Great Mystery with undying love, in order for your heart to fearlessly blossom into infinity and beyond."

The Protective Plant Mothers

The elder paused and looked at me, anticipating a question. I sighed, trying not to convey my frustration too volubly. I was stirred by the eloquence of his theory, but I had no idea how to apply it.

"Don Sinchi, you speak of Mother Nature in such abstract terms, but how do these inner human qualities relate to medicinal plants here in the rainforest that we just visited in your nursery? I want to understand how we might use practical methods to fulfill what you speak of, and I imagine the plants might help."

He replied, "The medicinal plants are also known by our people as 'mothers' and messengers of the Great Mystery, but in contrast to the Fierce Mothers of the dis-eases, who use our sickness to bring to our attention what we must learn and integrate, these mothers are protective. Plant spirits help the essential human qualities I just mentioned to become cultivated in you. The protective Plant Mothers nurture us as we solidify the evolutionary stepping-stones on our hero's journey.

"For example, if someone is working to overcome their fears, then Cedar bark can help instill the strength of spirit to face oneself. If someone has a lot of confusion, then a plant like Guayusa can help clear the mind. For sadness and depression, Passionflower is great. But the plants can truly help only once the issues at hand are consciously faced with honesty about one's shortcomings and remembrance of unconditional love. Otherwise, even the plants can become just another Band-Aid to cover festering wounds."

I admitted to Don Sinchi that I was still apprehensive about the Amazonian tradition because it was so different from the world I came from. It seemed too foreign and mysterious for my logical mind.

Don Sinchi replied softly, like a parent to a child, "Mystery is something one must form a relationship with on this path. If it weren't for your sickness, your path in life would've been quite ordinary. There are many well-walked paths in society, trodden by millions of people. All the steps, bends, and turns are already known on those mainstream toll roads of mundane existence, with no stone left unturned."

I laughed to myself. From my own experience in the modern world, I'd come to the same conclusion. "When everything is figured out for you, all that's left is a conveyor belt of obedience."

He grinned again and asked, "Isn't that the world of great scientific progress and achievements you come from, where through empirical and deductive methods, everything, at least in your immediate life, has been figured out for you? On the other hand, by coming here, to our primitive society, you chose to forge a new path, with a different direction—a much less-traveled path of self-discovery. A path like this will never be boring, since you are venturing into the infinite mystery of the heart's wisdom."

Tool: Restoration of Health

A Lupuna seed (which comes from a Kapok tree, whose seeds, leaves, bark, and resin are healing antidotes to disorders ranging from dysentery to kidney disease) must settle into the fertile ground in order to grow into a millennial tree giant. Similarly, we must immerse ourselves in the womb of Mother Nature's love and reveal all our shadows within her embrace. Only then can our healing potential be realized.

We often run from our shadows out of fear and ignorance. Consider the ways you deal with pain, discomfort, tensions, and unresolved issues in your life. Take a moment to consider an affliction you've lived with for some time. It might be mental, emotional, or physical (or a combination). Write down the many ways you've resisted this affliction.

Next, consider how you can embrace your dis-ease with the love of your entire being. Write down the many ways this affliction is a universal lesson of love waiting to be realized.

Whenever you become angry, impatient, or frustrated, return to both lists to recognize how your resistance is getting in the way of your healing. As Don Sinchi told me, on the path of evolutionary healing, everyone is responsible for sabotaging their health and also restoring it. But with intentional presence and a little help from Mother Nature, we can remember ourselves to be a small mystery within the Great Mystery of the universe.

Respecting Nature's Wisdom

Don Sinchi lit his pipe and loudly blew smoke over my stomach, exactly where my physical issue was located. While I was enveloped in smoke, the elder stood up and left me alone in the maloka.

Astounded by all that had just unfolded, I remained seated in the healing space of the maloka for a long time, experiencing a profound inner silence that flowed freely amid the steady stream of oscillating sounds from the rainforest.

After returning to my hut that night, unable to sleep, I lay awake pondering all that had transpired so far in this otherworldly realm. Reflecting on my terminal illness and remembering the years of agonizing pain before coming to the Amazon, I was determined to keep engaging the ancient healing discipline I'd found here. To heal at my very core, I had to understand what Don Sinchi meant about me being responsible for ruining my own health. While I recognized the truth in much of what he said, I found myself bristling at this idea. How could I be responsible when I had contracted my illness as a small child?

On the day of the next ceremony, Don Sinchi called me to the firepit near the maloka, where the Ayahuasca potion was being concocted. The elder referred to this place as his medicine kitchen. As I approached, he said, "Romancito, come sit with me while we prepare the medicine. It will help your connection with the plant spirit."

As I sat down on an old wood stump next to him, he added, "Watch the flow of the bubbles in the cauldron—the spirit of the medicine will connect to you through them."

I started to observe the hypnotic ripples of bubbles in the pot. Although the pot was boiling intensely, there seemed to be a pattern and order to the seeming chaos. It was as if the pot, the fire underneath, and the bubbling brew inside were all part of a living organism that was experiencing us in that very moment, just as we were experiencing it.

"How long do you boil this medicine, Don Sinchi?" I asked, stirred by the sensation of being watched.

"The fastest time I can prepare a good medicine is fourteen hours. But a really good, refined brew needs to be cooked for three days. These kinds of brews are used for special occasions, like a grave sickness or a reunion of elders. The process of cooking the medicine is a ceremony in and of itself. You will find out for yourself in due time when a deeper connection with this tradition develops. As you already know, there are two main teacher plants in this brew: the Ayahuasca vine and the Chakruna leaf. Sometimes I also put in Yage Huambisa, or Chaliponga Chakrapanga, as some tribes call it, as well as other plants that Spirit guides me to. Of course, we don't just throw the plants in the pot like you would noodles into hot water. The leaves need to be torn to bits, and the vine needs to be thoroughly broken down. Then we put the leaves and the vine in a specific order inside the pot and fill it with water, almost to the brim. I also have a special stone I put on top in order to add the powerful energy of Mother Earth to the concoction.

"For the medicine to be effective, it cannot be left unattended throughout the entire time of the cook. Whoever is overseeing the process keeps a dieta, or maintains *ayuno*, a state of fasting where only water or medicinal plant teas can be consumed. During the cook, the most important part is an intentional presence. That includes contemplating, praying, singing icaros, and concentrating—or meditating, as you may call it. As we deepen our relationship with this tradition, we begin to trust Mother Nature's wisdom within ourselves as well. One day, she will take you under her wing and start teaching you directly. Until then, you will have to listen to an old fool like me."

His eyes twinkled with laughter as he uttered the last sentence.

"By no means do I think you are a fool, Don Sinchi," I protested.

Don Sinchi measured me with his glistening eyes and said, "We are all fools. It's just that some of us already know this."

At that moment, Don Sinchi's nephew, Chispa, showed up to tell us a patient had come to see him. Don Sinchi commented that the Great Spirit had sent us a messenger to deliver an evolutionary lesson. The elder invited me to join him, and we left Chispa to tend to the medicine in our absence.

As we approached Don Sinchi's house, we saw a very overweight woman waiting for us. There was something unnatural about her. She moved, talked, and behaved as if her body were a marionette manipulated by an invisible hand. She told us that she lived in a nearby mestizo settlement and that for the past 15 years, she had not felt like herself. She was always tired and experienced pains in her belly, as well as constant hunger, no matter how much she ate. She had tried many pharmaceuticals, but they only made her feel worse to the point of desperation, which is why she'd finally decided to visit Don Sinchi.

The Rimyurá listened attentively to the woman's account; when she was done, he palpated her belly to observe her reactions. He then asked her to sit on a chair in front of him. He picked up his ceremonial *chakapa* (a healing instrument used by curanderos, assembled from the leaves of a small brush plant) and began to whistle. As soon as he stopped chanting and blew the mapacho smoke over her belly, the woman started screaming that she felt something moving inside her. The next thing we knew, a three-foot-long black worm slithered out from under her dress. Don Sinchi immediately squished it on the ground with his foot. He then looked at the frightened woman and calmly told her that she had a case of intestinal worm possession. The elder added that there were a few more of them living inside her, but she shouldn't worry because she'd come to the right place.

He proceeded to ask her a few questions about her recent diet. The woman responded that she hadn't eaten anything that day because of tremendous discomfort following anything she put in her mouth. Listening to the patient with a concerned face, he told her to lie down in the hammock and join us in the ceremony later that evening.

We then returned to the medicine kitchen near the maloka to continue with the medicine cook. I was perplexed by what had happened to the poor woman, but all Don Sinchi told me was that he'd invoked his healing plant spirits, who'd helped the woman's body expel a worm.

"The rest we will find out in tonight's ceremony," he tersely commented.

As the presence of the Ayahuasca spirit evaporating through the steam rising from the pot enveloped us, I became curious about the plant spirits Don Sinchi had mentioned. I shared with him that many people view the ingestion of medicinal plants in terms of how helpful their bio-phytochemical components will be to the human organism. He laughed and said that with this kind of view, it would be impossible to heal the source of suffering in people's lives.

Don Sinchi then pointed to the rainforest around us. "In this place, each plant has its own spirit. By establishing a relationship with the plant spirits, their healing effects can be magnified a thousandfold. As the connection with plant spirits deepens, there may no longer be a need to ingest the plants anymore. The plant spirits can then be invoked at will for one's own healing first, and eventually, for that of others. Each plant spirit is a key that unlocks our natural potential for well-being."

From my personal experience, I knew he was right about the difficulty of recovering from sickness in today's world. Modern society feeds an insatiable multitrillion-dollar health-care industry. It helps people just enough for them to become dependent on it and keep paying for treatments without any hope of complete recovery. Modern medicine and pharmaceutical companies take advantage of Mother Nature for petty, egotistical gains.

Just then, something clicked into place for me. My eyes widened as I considered the ways in which big pharma manipulates the human organism as it would a machine, destroying the spirit of Nature through its extraction of active ingredients from the plants and copyrighting them for the sake of profit. For every symptom that is resolved in this way, several others manifest. Then, reputable doctors prescribe other pills for all the side effects that come up, creating a complete dependency in the mainstream population. As a result, people come out of pharmacies with shopping bags full of "medicine." This consumption perpetuates and increases as time passes, for the rest of their lives.

As I shared all this with Don Sinchi, he suddenly became serious. "Each plant speaks the language of nature. Modern pills are just a jumbled-up pile of letters that make no sense to the human body. This problem goes even deeper. I know many people who've forgotten their connection to Mother Nature, even though they still live in the rainforest. For example, the patient we just saw is a pawn of the corrupt mentality that rules the world today, by making people forget the wisdom of nature within and all around them. When these people get sick, instead of using the miraculous healing powers of plants, they and their families cut down the trees, burn them, and sell them as charcoal in the city. Charcoal is a popular commodity in the rainforest, used for cooking and export. The money made from such a scheme is used to buy pharmaceuticals from barefoot doctors in Iquitos—street vendors who sell pharmaceutical drugs without a prescription—who cause even more health problems with their pills. One of those burned trees could have helped many people get well without any alternative agenda of egocentric profit. Nowadays, not only do people forget their essential true nature, but they also destroy all possible reminders of Nature around them."

I considered the question that had troubled me so deeply the night before. I'd struggled with the idea that I was responsible for having "ruined" my health, considering I'd developed my illness at such a young age. But now, I was beginning to understand that Don Sinchi's words were not ones of blame. Rather, he was helping me understand that I'd been born into a set of conditions that were ubiquitous in the Western world. I'd been born and raised in a society and culture that had zapped Mother Nature's medicine of its sacredness. It wasn't my fault that the proverbial wool had been pulled over my eyes, as this was true for a vast majority of humans . . . but it was my responsibility to rip the veil of ignorance away, so I could step back into my true nature.

Tool: The Right Use of Creativity

How have you dishonored the seeds of nature within you? Recognize any ways in which you have used your creativity in the past to avoid the issues or find a quick fix. For example, it's possible to be creative when it comes to finding a variety of instant gratifications, just so you don't have to face discomfort. You might also find yourself inventing different reasons just so you don't have to deal with a difficult task at hand. How can you engage your creativity as a discipline that provides long-term, lasting transformation? Come up with at least three different creative tools for learning to confront discomfort. You may be surprised at what you find! Regardless, be sure to implement these methods on a regular basis and observe the results.

Essential Links in the Spiral of Life

Don Sinchi took a pause, lit his pipe, and blew smoke into the boiling cauldron that held the medicine. He then added almost silently, "The rainforest is suffering, Mother Earth is suffering, and people are suffering. It was not always like that and will not remain this way for long. Pacha Mama is patient, but not stupid. Her awakening power will soon emerge from the luminous core of the underworld to teach all of humanity a big lesson in humility."

I asked Don Sinchi to clarify what he meant by the "underworld." He replied, "The shadow realm is where the seeds of life are planted and our greatest potential is gestated. Although we humans forget that we are a part of Nature and try to hide in our rational minds, the Great Mother is always here to remind us of our connection with her. She is always under our very feet, supporting us on our journey toward the higher self.

"In our Yahua tradition, there are two levels to the underworld. The first level of the shadow dimension is a superficial one, where we bury all our unresolved issues and unprocessed emotional energies. We do so by being consumers, endlessly taking from our Mother without caring for her and the rest of her creation.

"The second level is related to the tremors and impulses of our deepest unconscious behavior; they are in control of our lives without us even realizing it.

"The power of instinctual urges is uncontainable and can cause much suffering to oneself and others, unless channeled through a heart-centered awareness. Pacha Mama, the Mother of the World, must get strict with her children when they become spoiled brats and forget to honor the seeds of their heart's wisdom. The plant spirits remind us to nurture the seeds of unconditional love, which Nature planted in us as well. We can tune in to the luminous core of the Great Mother by remembering to listen to the rhythm of our own heartbeat."

Don Sinchi paused and looked at the rainforest around us with deep reverence. The steam rising from the pot was blurring my eyesight, and all I could see were the many shades of green merging into a vibrant unity. The elder also became blurry, but he gradually came back into focus.

He continued: "The health of the rainforest depends on the interconnectedness of all life within it. The roots of the plants are where the synergy of life begins. Mother Earth unconditionally supports the circle of life. Genuine relatedness begins from the very roots of our existence. All the challenges, wounds, struggles, and aspirations together create the fertile ground of our shadow realm. In fact, genuine relatedness sprouts in the underworld. Our wish is to be entirely free in our hearts so that we can embody the love that never dies. The real practice begins when we sincerely share that wish with ourselves and each other, as a way to make it a constant reality. When the plant spirits are approached with pure intentions, they help remind us that all beings share that wish, but out of ignorance, they don't see the forest behind the trees. Without seeing how we are all related through our struggles to find happiness, we end up hurting ourselves and each other."

"So, who are these plant spirits, Don Sinchi? Are they external entities of some kind?" I asked.

Don Sinchi raised an eyebrow. "Either you are pulling my Yahua tail right now, or your inner eye is still shut very tightly. Nevertheless, I will tell you.

"Since we are all living organisms and the same organic intelligence has created all of us, each of Nature's creations reflects the rest. The plant spirits embody essential characteristics of the Great Spirit that can help us recognize these same enlightened qualities in ourselves and others. The healing spirits of Nature are therefore referred to as *doctorcitos* in our culture. Their qualities sustain the dynamic equilibrium of our organism, making physical healing possible.

"There is always an emotional root of imbalance to every disease. The dis-ease of forgetfulness I keep telling you about can manifest in a multitude of ways. Separation from nature can occur through fear, confusion, obsessiveness, arrogance, or anger, among many others. While there are many expressions of suffering, they can all be traced back to the same trap of self-absorption plaguing today's civilization."

I couldn't help but interject. "Don Sinchi, please tell me how I can heal the root of suffering and be free from the trap of self-absorption!"

"To liberate yourself from the trap of self-obsession, you must learn to see through appearances. Everything is interconnected—this is the cornerstone of our living wisdom tradition. The Great Spirit is not an abstract thing, but more real than this material world, which also includes our physical bodies. *Nothing is possible without everything.* We are all essential links in the spiral of life. Whether we know it or not, we are always in service of the Great Spirit that ushers a myriad of life-forms into existence. Everything comes and goes, everyone is born, and everyone dies, but life itself is eternal and perpetual. The ancients discovered that the Great Spirit of Love consists of each of our spirits individually and is reflected back to us simultaneously by a universe filled with mirrorlike wisdom. All our passions, inspirations, and whatever else each of us lives for mirrors the greater energy flow in the world at large."

Don Sinchi explained that his ancestors referred to the Great Spirit as the higher consciousness of Nature, which allows Nature's majesty to be experienced directly, both within and without. The rainforest, as a multifaceted expression of Nature's intelligence, can help us discover the wisdom of our own bodies, which are also Nature. Of course, we humans get stuck in our heads and forget that we are Nature. The ancestors recognized that the plants were a gift to humanity, corresponding to specific qualities and values that would help us embody the full glory of our collective spirit. Don Sinchi explained that we must keep engaging consistently and wholeheartedly with every moment of life, in order to transform our foolishness and recognize that we are all connected.

When the Rimyurá stopped talking, we sat in silence, observing the numerous tiny bubbles, all perfectly in sync with one another as they formed magnificent designs in the boiling cauldron of Ayahuasca.

My conversation with the elder only amplified a feeling that had grown in me ever since arriving in the Amazon: I sensed that we were at a critical threshold in human and planetary history.

Spending time with the Yahua elder, while preparing the sacred medicine and speaking candidly about the state of the world, felt like medicine for the soul. Through Don Sinchi, I could see the profound wisdom of the ancient Amazonian people.

I sat there by the fire next to Don Sinchi, while he whistled incantations and sang icaros until the sacrament was properly cooked. Once we were done, there was only enough time for me to jump into a creek and wash off the sweat before the start of the ceremony. Refreshed by my swim, I headed back into the maloka, eager for what would arise in the next ceremony.

REFLECTIONS

- My frustration with Don Sinchi's tendency to share information that felt confusing to my logical mind or that lacked practical application gradually gave way to a deeper understanding: there is another type of knowledge that is not logical or conceptual, but that is about the embodiment of well-being. My logical mind was simply not effective when it came to processing Nature's higher intelligence. An essential step on the path of initiation is the willingness to stop trying to comprehend everything with the mind. *How are you engaging with the information in this book? Are you attempting to understand everything with your logical mind? Is it possible for you to instead engage with the poetic senses of the heart?*

- With the sincere wish to resolve an obvious suffering in my life, I was bent on discovering the depth and wisdom of Don Sinchi's Evolutionary Science. The more I learned about myself, the more I realized the depth of my ignorance. *On your own spiritual journey, where have you come directly into contact with your ignorance? Did this discourage you, or did it help you tap into a deeper source of motivation? How can cultivating humility help you persevere on your own path?*

- Although I initially struggled with the idea that I was responsible for my illness, which I'd contracted at a young age, I came to recognize that the conditions of the society I'd been raised in had planted seeds of ignorance that kept me from seeing reality as it is. I stopped blaming myself and became more proactive in finding sources of healing. *How is blame different from accountability? Where are you blaming yourself instead of taking genuine accountability for your own afflictions?*

- Although the dogma of Western society might lead to misperceptions about the underworld, Don Sinchi explained to me that the underworld is where our greatest potential is gestated. It is where we come to recognize our intrinsic connection with our true nature and with the Great Mother. *What is your relationship to the underworld? What do you think of when you see that word? In what ways might traveling into the shadow realm help you reconnect with truth?*

- Don Sinchi shared five pathologies that emerge from cultivating the seeds of unhelpful emotions and tendencies. These lead to ignorance, which leads to suffering. *Reflect on the five main pathologies on page 61 and the three unconscious tendencies of ignorance, craving, and aversion. In what ways have these manifested in your life? How have you consciously or unconsciously allowed them to proliferate and dictate your experience of your health and your overall reality?*

- Without seeing how we are all related through our struggles to find happiness, we end up hurting ourselves and each other instead. But in the words of Don Sinchi, "Nothing is possible without everything." *What is your experience of feeling the interconnectedness of all beings? How do you continue to separate yourself from others, especially those toward whom you feel judgment? What would it take, and what would it look like, to invite greater connection?*

CHAPTER 5

THE SECOND CEREMONY

Understanding Demons

The second ceremony brought me into the depths of my fears and inhibitions.

The medicine started working on me right after Don Sinchi's initial invocations, and I received a vivid vision of an exquisite mandala wheel embedded with an intricate design from the Tibetan tradition that I had previously seen photos of. This mandala, however, was alive and breathing with brilliant colors. The iridescent images within the wheel, accompanied by its pulsating expansion and contraction, were in sync with the rhythm of my breath.

I became consumed by the marvelous mirage, knowing that the only reason it could be so in sync with me was that it reflected my own energetic state. I remembered Don Sinchi's words about humans' deeper nature. Experiencing with crystal clarity the brilliant mandala in my entire field of vision, I felt it with my entire being. The only detail about the mandala that was not clear was the very center of it, which appeared hazy, with dark shapes chaotically moving within it. With increased focus, I zoomed into the core of the marvel I was witnessing. The center of the mandala became amplified . . . and the next thing I knew, I was being propelled into it.

I felt like I was teleported into another dimension and had ended up in what felt like a deep underground cave. I couldn't see anything, but I could hear hissing and swishing sounds all around me. Although my five senses told me I was in another dimension, there was a sixth sense maintaining a vague connection to the maloka in the earthly realm. When Don Sinchi lit his sacred pipe in the temple, I saw the darkness of the otherworldly cave illuminated as well. What I saw horrified me to my bones: this underground cave was actually a pit full of vipers. The realization that right in the center of the most exquisite mandala was such a hideous place only added to my horror.

Countless twisting, intertwining, squirming serpents completely surrounded me. The vipers were everywhere, and there was no way out. They came closer and closer until I was totally overrun. In that moment, some mysterious power came along and whisked me away, transplanting me back in the maloka. Once I was fully back in my body, I purged intensely and uncontrollably all over myself and the sacred ground of our sanctum. I was covered in cold sweat and slimy vomit, but I was ecstatic to be alive and out of the viper pit.

It was at that point in the ceremony that Don Sinchi's ill, overweight patient began releasing another parasite, as she screamed at the top of her lungs. Throughout the night, the poor woman ended up releasing four tremendous worms altogether amid the most chilling screams. Calmly, Don Sinchi squished all of them underfoot, while blowing protective smoke from his pipe on the woman and everyone else in the room.

Although I was still facing the depths of my own darkness, I was not as agitated as I had been in the previous ceremony. I had begun to develop a greater trust in Mother Nature and her medicine!

Don Sinchi told us throughout the ceremony that many demons were leaving the magical protection circle. At one point during that ceremony, the head of a terrifying monster the size of a house appeared in front of me. Its face shifted and moved in the same manner as the vipers in the pit. My first reaction was to recoil and look away, but Don Sinchi started speaking to someone he was healing at that moment . . . and somehow, his words related directly to my experience.

I heard Don Sinchi say with a chuckle, "Oye, don't run away from the things that you are fearful of, you hear? Hating the monsters only turns you into another monster."

These words reignited my intuitive connection with the medicine, with the medicine man, and with the healing circle. It became clearer to me why this was a healing ceremony and how I could more consciously support my own and others' process. I was guided to maintain a steady gaze on my monster without judging or classifying it in any way. After a few moments that seemed like an eternity, the apparition suddenly transformed into a bouquet of beautiful, rainbow-colored flowers that bloomed over my entire field of vision.

It occurred to me that the Goddess of Nature was hiding inside this scary monster! I finally understood: she was truly a loving mother who had to be strict in order to shake all that was not natural out of my body, mind, and spirit. My continuous practice was to keep allowing the powerful vibration of her life force to stream through my being. Cradled within the womb of the Goddess, which the temple floor seemed to have transformed into, I eventually fell asleep.

Getting to Know the Monsters

Upon waking inside the maloka in the morning, I went to bathe in the creek before I sought out Don Sinchi. I found him by the medicine kitchen, chopping wood. Seeing me, he put down the ax and invited me to sit with him as he took time to rest. Once I settled in, I asked him to clarify what he'd meant about demons leaving the circle during last night's healing session.

He explained that when the spirit of Mother Nature descends into the ceremony, it's subtle yet infinitely stronger than the dense, but only seemingly overwhelming, power of disruptive illusions—like the one I'd had of the viper pit. Once the two meet, the inner darkness of ignorance cannot hold the light of Universal Consciousness and instantly dissolves. For this reason, it's essential to stay within the healing circle throughout the ceremony: to help stabilize the light of Nature within.

"So, who are these monsters you talk about and where do they come from?" I asked.

"In our tribe, we have a saying: 'If you hate the monsters, then you are just another monster—and that's why they come to hang out with you.' Essentially, these demons are the result of unconscious reactions that turn into negative habits we develop to cope with challenging circumstances in life. Repeated long enough, they eventually form into behavioral patterns."

As I came to understand, the demons have their own evolutionary journey. If they are allowed to keep festering in the darkness of our ignorance, they eventually develop into autonomous personality constructs that imprison and exploit humanity's life force—just as the meat industry today does to farm animals. These artificial personality constructs impose restrictions on our lives through a fear-based mentality. People then seek protection from uncertainty and insecurity, simply because they don't trust the capacity of the heart to remain open with all the ups and downs of life.

I shared my vision of the mandala with Don Sinchi, and how the core of it had scared the hell out of me.

The Rimyurá nodded and said, "The healing circle of Mother Nature will hold space for you to face and transform your fears as she aids you with her unconditional love. You see, Romancito, out of fear, we sacrifice the freedom of aliveness in exchange for a comfortable yet numbing existence. You wear protective armor long enough, and eventually you become defined by it. This constrictive personality shell begins to dictate your life, as you mechanically keep reenacting the same behavior. The real protection, however, is openness and heart-centered presence. Desperately resisting life, while demanding that the world revolve around us, turns us into creatures of habit. Then, we constantly end up sitting on the thorny plants that we ourselves have unwittingly planted, without even realizing it. Because of these habitual patterns of resistance, the rivers of energy in our bodies become stagnant and distorted, causing dis-ease. The parasites form from these wriggling knots of energy that appeared to you at the very core of your true nature.

"These usual suspects then gather so much momentum that they begin generating their own parasitic consciousness. They can then make us do things against our will. Most people in the world lose monumental amounts of life energy to useless behavior that serves no one, aside from that parasitic consciousness. Now, if you yourself don't trust that love is the only reality at the very core of your being, who else do you think will settle there?

"Finally, these energetic parasites can actually attract physical entities—for example, intestinal worms—that embody these noncorporeal beings as they get stronger. If you keep harboring creatures that steal your awareness and do nothing about it, you eventually become totally enslaved by these monsters. Further down, they can even transfer your life force to their superiors, who are ancient demons that have been in existence for a long time, feeding on the unawareness of humankind. Those kinds of situations require an exorcism. The healing of the woman with parasites last night was an example of a light exorcism."

"So, the monsters are real!" I exclaimed.

Don Sinchi looked at me sternly, responding, "Let me ask you, Romancito, why have you hesitated to tell me about the illness you carry?"

I thought for a moment, surprised by the question, before answering: "Because of all the times I was ostracized due to my condition. I was met with pity, repulsion, or malevolence by people who knew about my illness."

Don Sinchi lit his pipe, and after puffing it for a good moment, commented: "When survival instinct becomes the main ruling power over one's life, it turns into a great monster. You see, Romancito, we make these monsters 'real' by feeding them with our unconscious behavior, which includes superstition and over-mystification.

"Many believe that ignorance is bliss and blame all their misfortunes on figments of their imagination. That habit of being triggered by everything turns people into slaves of their own monstrous behavior. However, these monsters are *not* the evil demonic entities they are often portrayed as. They're more like universal functions designed to take advantage of unused energy. These functions are imprints or empty molds that only get activated when they're filled with psychic energy that we leak. If we consciously channel our life force for a higher purpose, we start to attract *doctorcito* spirits, who represent the enlightened qualities of heart-centered awareness.

"Whether we attract enlightened or unenlightened spirits is based on how we utilize the awareness given to us by the higher consciousness of the Great Spirit. For our ancestors, every inch of this universe must be imbued with purpose. Our lives are heroic acts of directing our life force so we can embody a purpose greater than our individual selves. If our effort is lacking, we deteriorate. However, we still serve a higher purpose by becoming fertile ground for new life to be born."

I responded that, before coming to the Amazon, I'd worked in the corporate world, dedicating my energy to something that had no sense or meaning to me, except continuous subsistence in a consumerist reality. Everything Don Sinchi was telling me validated my own previously unnamed feeling that I'd just been feeding an insatiable system that uses human energy to destroy life on the planet . . . all for the sake of a momentary illusion of happiness.

Don Sinchi nodded. "What our ancestors referred to as the eternal struggle between the light and dark forces comes down to the wisdom of truth versus the ignorance of distraction. There's your freedom of choice: you can consciously choose to be useful, as a conduit of Universal Love, or you can be useless and unconscious—in which case Universal Love will make useful compost out of you.

"Once the entire human race voluntarily submits its will to the monster of self-absorption, the evolution of our species will end. Then, there will be no more sense for us to keep dragging out such a miserable existence. When that happens, we'd better vacate the premises for other species to have better luck than us! But, as long as at least one human being can maintain awareness of fearless love as a state of ultimate health, the rest of us still have a chance. The indestructible truth of who we are can only be found in the wisdom of interconnectedness. It's our own ignorance that is worse than any external monster."

The Truth behind Truth

Captivated by his explanation, I asked him something that had been on my mind for a while. "How would you define truth, Don Sinchi?"

The Rimyurá thought for a second. Although the elder's body became very still, his presence beamed with aliveness and seemed all-encompassing. As he spoke, he deliberately chose his words while fixing his gaze beyond the horizon that was hidden from ordinary human eyes by the dense rainforest.

"It has been my experience that truth is beyond words and description. Truth is not a concept or an idea, but a state of being. We can all recognize it in ourselves and each other beyond all doubts because it's deeply anchored in love and compassion for all beings. Each of us experienced such love in the womb. None of us would be born and stay alive without it.

"A truthful state can dispel the greatest gloom by shining like the light of a thousand suns. Even a glimpse of it can dissolve ignorance. All I can do is merely point toward that essence within us all, but I can never fully explain it. That essence can only be experienced directly with humility, receptivity, and the readiness to honestly face everything that stands in the way."

We both remained silent for a while, with only the chirping of the birds and the humming of the insects accompanying us. Yet, despite all the profound insights and the post-ceremony afterglow, I was distracted by physical hunger.

Don Sinchi exhaled loudly and got up to go back toward the maloka. I followed the elder; once we were inside, he handed me a rake. Don Sinchi pointed to my purge on the sandy floor, as well as the stains from the squished intestinal worms from the night before. He said, "Cleaning up after your mess and helping clean the mess of others is an essential part of the healing journey—not just on the physical level, but also the energetic one. The more effectively you can clean up after yourself, the better you can assimilate the essential evolutionary insights as nutrients for your well-being. How's that going for you, by the way?"

I began to rake the purged-over sand, imagining it to be the Amazonian version of Japanese Zen gardening. "Although I try, it's been hard for me to focus on these profound topics that you share, Don Sinchi, with my stomach rumbling from the bland dieta food. I can't help but crave all kinds of foods that I used to enjoy in the past, but which are forbidden in my dieta, like hamburgers and pizza."

The Rimyurá laughed, saying, "These are your parasite monsters speaking right now! They are never happy about the dieta and like to throw pity parties once in a while. Especially when the profound meaning of life is being revealed, nothing seems more real than hamburgers and pizza!"

The healer winked at me with a spark in his eyes and continued with a more serious expression: "Also, you should know that during the healing process, it's common to crave what your organism is detoxing. Our healing tradition is about learning to honor the truth of your being, above all the pleasure senses. The dieta is a symbol that allows us to contemplate the focus of our intentions in this life. Only by seeing more clearly than ever all the coping mechanisms and habits of avoidance that rule your life can you begin to transform them."

I retorted that I didn't know how to begin, because I was still struggling to comprehend the teachings of the Amazonian ancestors.

"What I've been sharing with you so far was not directed toward your mind. To simplify, you can relate to it this way: if you jump a lot from one explanation to another without taking the time to see how it relates to the truth of your being, you will eventually get a head the size of a watermelon and a heart the size of a cashew."

Don Sinchi took a few puffs of his pipe, and after blowing the smoke all over my body, said, "Humanity's accumulated wisdom stretches back to beginningless time. To keep it from being diluted, it was guarded with great secrecy from generation to generation and made available to very few, select individuals. In ancient times, however, even those fortunate few were restricted to the perspective of their geographic location. That made the journey of awakening even more difficult."

I thought about how many ancient wisdom lineages had converged into the melting pot of our technologically interconnected world. You could find spiritual teachings on the Internet or fly to all kinds of exotic locations. But from what I'd learned in the Amazon, it was essential to get to know one specific path deep enough first, in order to directly experience the universal truth it pointed to. With an embodied perspective, I could begin to recognize the same truth of being within other spiritual paths as well.

Don Sinchi continued, "The experiential approach of Amazonian sorcery was always meant for the realization of our true nature as the source of evolutionary healing. Amazonian curanderos are also referred to as *curiosos*, or the curious ones, here in the rainforest—because curiosity is essential to finding a cure. There are glorious legends that still remain of our ancestors' curiosity being intertwined with practical, earth-based spirituality. They discovered their highest potential by vulnerably sharing with and learning from other tribes, and even distant kingdoms, what it means to be alive. I would daresay that the cornerstone of all ancient cultures is realizing the truth as a state of inner peace and well-being so we can share it with our fellow humans everywhere. No tradition in the world has a monopoly on truth. The only absolute truth is that there *is* no absolute truth. Everything and everyone is relative to each other and are relatives of each other."

The elder finished his account by lighting his pipe once more and blowing smoke all around the maloka. As he spoke these final words, I was propelled into a forgotten and mysterious realm, filled with the magic of infinite possibilities for all the ways human civilization could flourish. Don Sinchi however, declined to discuss his tradition further with me that day, saying that I had heard enough and there was no sense indulging in chitchat if I didn't take time to be with myself and apply what had been shared to my direct experience. He told me to go back to my hut and stay there in isolation until further notice.

I took his reluctance to chew up all the information for me to be similar to the koan riddles offered by Zen monks to their disciples. Instead of expecting all the answers to be instantly provided, I had to sit with my teacher's explanations. To get to the deeper layers of meaning, I had to make the context relevant to my own experience.

As I settled into my hut for the night, my head and heart were swimming in revelations. Slowly but surely, I was awakening from the dream of separation! With that thought, I fell asleep.

Tool: Knowing Your Monsters

Get to know your inner conflicts, fears, inhibitions, and the unconscious patterns of reactivity in your life. What are your triggers? What situations in your life provoke disturbances in you? The more you are aware of your unconscious patterns and the circumstances that encourage them, the less likely you are to be caught by surprise and get trapped in doing the same thing over and over again, while expecting a different result (Einstein's definition of insanity). Develop a strategy to apply the essential human qualities from the tool kit you created from previous chapters, especially in moments of turmoil.

"Sharlamans" and Amazonian Sorcerers

A few days later, Don Sinchi showed up at my hut early in the morning and invited me to join him on a trip into the jungle to collect the plant medicines necessary to prepare Ayahuasca. He said that Ayahuasca had gotten to know me enough in the previous ceremonies to permit a visitation of her habitat. The Rimyurá performed an initiatory ritual by blowing smoke on me from his pipe for cleansing and protection. While I was enveloped in the smoke, he sang various icaros I had heard him sing in previous ceremonies. Upon finishing, Don Sinchi said, "In order not to break my protective spell, you must be totally silent and as quiet as possible with your steps while walking through the forest. This ritual was done for you to sustain pure intentions, so as not to disturb Nature's guardian spirits with your mental chatter as you step on the medicine path."

I quietly followed the footsteps of the medicine man deep into the rainforest on an almost invisible trail, surrounded by a dense wall of foliage on each side. After an hour or so, we came into an open meadow encircled by immense trees growing at a distance from each other. Right away, the Ayahuasca spirit called my attention, and I saw her thick vines lovingly wrapping themselves around tremendous tree giants. The sun was brightly illuminating everything around us to the point that I had to squint my eyes.

Don Sinchi leaned in and uttered, "Ayahuasca is somewhat contradictory about her growing conditions—she likes the sun and the shade of big, tall trees simultaneously. Her nature is of the Earth and deep roots; however, she reaches for the sun with the embrace of her vines.

"Reaching toward Father Sun, plants must be careful, for they can easily dry out without a shady umbrella of leaves to protect them and the deep roots to nurture them with fresh water. Same with us humans—without the balance of all the essential spiritual elements, our life energy cannot rise to its greatest evolutionary potential. If our current civilization flies too close to Father Sun without honoring what he represents in relation to all the other elemental qualities within each being, we are doomed. All the expressions of Mother Nature must be equally honored for life to continue.

"Ayahuasca teaches us to engage with the forces of nature skillfully and responsibly, so that we can be of benefit to the world and not harm ourselves or others."

Don Sinchi reached into his bag and pulled out a handful of loose mapacho leaves. He whistled into the tobacco in his fist and then buried it next to the Mother Vine as an offering. The elder then grasped the vine with both hands, while saying a prayer in the Yahua language. Upon finishing the prayer, we both stood still for a few minutes, letting the prayer connect with the spirit of the plant.

After some time, the Rimyurá retrieved a machete from his satchel and matter-of-factly began to chop the vine with it. We hid the bag with Ayahuasca cuttings in the bushes nearby, to pick up on the way back, and continued walking into the wilderness. We walked for about an hour more into the rainforest and finally came into a grove of Chakruna and Chaliponga trees. We stood there for some time, absorbing the serene and enchanting ambience of the sacred plants, and then proceeded to carefully collect a few small bags of the leaves from the trees. Once we were done, we bowed down to the plant spirits, expressing gratitude and leaving loose mapacho leaves for them in exchange. Then, we began our meditative silent walk back toward the house to start the cooking process.

As we trailed the rainforest, I couldn't help but think to myself how the healing tradition is so much more than just the ingestion of the substance. The humid air, sounds of the birds and animals, smells of aromatic flowers and decomposing stale foliage, and hum of Nature's life force were all essential to the medicine. The cumulative insights of the ancestors into the nature of reality, gathered by countless generations, were also an integral part of this ecosystem.

Don Sinchi smiled as I shared my reflection. He said, "The essence of Amazonian culture is an immeasurable treasure that cannot be counterfeited. The wisdom of the ancestors can only be embodied by real people, who in turn encourage others to keep putting it to the test of their personal life experience."

Back at the medicine kitchen, as we broke down the vine into tiny threads with the elder's "baseball bats," the Rimyurá told me, "Get ready for your next meeting with the Goddess tonight. In our tradition of Ayahuasca, it's essential to go through at least three ceremonies in a two-week period for a thorough cleanse and an initiation into the magnificent realm of the Great Spirit. Until you go through this initiation with an experienced and trustworthy shaman who can oversee your transformation, you will not be ready to hear or understand her guidance."

Don Sinchi's words brought up something that had been on my mind. I said, "I have been here in the Amazon for a few months now and have seen quite a few medicine men and women.

However, I've never heard anything like what you shared with me thus far from any of them. Neither have I witnessed the level of sobriety and lucid presence you seem to emanate with your whole being, Don Sinchi. Mostly, I have only heard mystical and superstitious inanities from belligerent 'shamans.' Why is that?"

He gave me a sad smile. "Unfortunately, most of my peers today are lost in the aberrations of their personal fantasies. So much has happened to our people since the time when Evolutionary Science was whole and complete. Today, you will mostly find tiny fragments of the original perspective here and there. I have dedicated a lifetime to collecting them, and I still have only few and far between. Sadly, the priorities of the modern world are more about the quantity of entertainment rather than the quality of realization."

Don Sinchi gave a contemptuous snort and said, "Some of them perform grandiose shows, and yet, what they provide is just that: a theatrical display that might wow someone who doesn't know better, but ultimately will have no effect on the evolution of consciousness. Many people, both local and foreign, after studying with these 'sharlamans' for long periods of time, are embarrassed to admit to themselves that they wasted many years in vain. They often defend what they do by spreading overly mystical and confusing worldviews to others."

I asked him what he meant by "overly mystical and confusing worldviews."

He chuckled. "I am referring to a misguided belief system that many of my colleagues live by today. The idea of external forces and spirits, which are separate from oneself, is based on a false perspective. Although the pictures these sharlamans paint appeal to many, their pseudo-animistic view is quite disempowering. Our ancestors' enlightened perspective points out how all external forces relate to the inner processes of evolutionary healing. Without the authentic guidance of a living wisdom lineage, it's easy to become a slave to external conditions, to the point that we see them as having power over us.

"The mirrorlike wisdom of the ancestors was all about an empowering view, where outer circumstances are transformed by inner qualities. That is the miraculous gift the original Evolutionary Science blessed humanity with. The primordial epoch in which this was revealed gave birth to human civilization all across the world. Unfortunately, nowadays this insight that the outer world merely reflects our inner mental and emotional states has become something many are oblivious to."

Don Sinchi went on to explain, however, that among these sharlamans there still exist some sorcerers (although they are few and far between) who are capable of harnessing the powerful forces of Nature. They have access to formidable energies, and some abilities when it comes to genuine manifestation—but, lacking a pure heart, they too get lost in self-absorbed agendas. These individuals end up even more miserable than most people for abusing their sacred gifts for selfish purposes.

"Access to the great powers of Mother Nature entails great responsibility," Don Sinchi said. "Those who intentionally hurt others for instant gratification, fame, and riches reap the suffering they sow many times over. Intentionally working to benefit all beings is the real purpose upon which our wisdom is based. Those who have no respect for the wise ancestors who initiated the Amazonian sacred plant traditions are commonly referred to as *brujos* here. Although some brujos have superficial and fleeting triumphs, inevitably, their deeds catch up with them. The misuse of Mother Nature's uncontainable life force has a shattering effect on their fragile egos. Sooner or later, all brujos face one of three fates: debilitating illness, raving madness, or a torturous death. In our Evolutionary Science, this is known as a protective mechanism.

"Called *cutipa* in Kichwa, this term was inaccurately translated into Spanish as *castigo* (punishment). In reality, of course, these black magicians castigate themselves with their own ignorance. Cutipa is a safety mechanism built into Evolutionary Science by the ancients, to prevent those who lack pure intentions from accessing greater powers on this path. Unfortunately, in their quest to satisfy their greed and superficial desires, these fools often end up harming many gullible, unaware people."

Don Sinchi went on to share that there is an even smaller percentage of practitioners who are known to be legitimate curanderos. They work from their hearts with a sincere dedication to awaken the healing potential of all beings around them. They also have the ability to consciously channel advanced universal states to alleviate suffering in those who are not yet ready to awaken their own inner healers.

"Regrettably, since the Amazonian region is being increasingly infested by the superficial values of modernity, even these genuine healers end up struggling with the consumerist mentality," Don Sinchi went on. "Having no social support for engaging the deeper meaning of our tradition, they end up drawing a line in their development. The demands of living in modern society take their toll. It's already hard enough to plant the seeds of evolution in the city mentality, which is cemented with fake values. For these seeds to sprout into absolute freedom from suffering is a monumental task. Yet, even in the noisiest and most polluted parts of Iquitos, I still find an occasional gem of Nature's resilience breaking through the concrete of ignorance. In today's world, there is a tiny percentage of people who remain among the final category of sorcerers. Those are the ones who have retained the blueprint of the original Evolutionary Science, alongside the pure intention to make it a reality."

Don Sinchi explained that in ancient times, people recognized these evolutionary healers as sorcerers of the highest degree and called them the *Banco Muraya*. Such people are not interested in publicity and either live unnoticed in society or hide deep in the jungle. In either case, Banco Murayas are almost impossible to find these days. They are the only curanderos who not only heal but also recover the spirit of the patient. They help people find their way to their full potential in the realm of never-ending possibilities.

Don Sinchi stopped talking at this point, and we sat quietly for some time. When I finally decided to comment on what he'd shared, the elder stopped me by raising his hand in the air. He told me we had spoken enough, and it was time for him to focus on whistling icaros and blowing the mapacho smoke into the medicine pot.

We continued to cook the medicine for many hours under the blazing heat of the fire, which required constant care. Just being in the presence of the steamy Ayahuasca vapors was making it hard for me to think straight. Many times throughout the cook, I felt as if the medicine was already working inside me. Don Sinchi's icaros helped tremendously, and I was surprised by how receptive I was to the melodies, even without drinking the sacrament. I shared with him that I felt myself experiencing the effects of Ayahuasca just from breathing the steam from the pot. He nodded and said that my receptivity was a good sign, signifying that my relationship with Mother Ayahuasca was deepening.

We cooked the medicine late into the night. There was no time to rest afterward, even though I wanted to. Instead, I took a dunk in the creek and went straight into the maloka. Don Sinchi also washed himself and arrived at the ceremonial circle shortly after me with a freshly prepared batch of the sacred plant medicine.

Tool: Developing Spiritual Discernment

Have you ever met or known a sharlaman? How do you know whether someone is engaging in spiritual bypassing? What is their belief system and ideology?

Especially when sacred plant ceremonies are concerned, working with the psyche is a delicate process that can be compared to energetic brain surgery. Do you want a qualified brain surgeon or a mere lobotomist to work with you? Other questions to ask yourself about whether you've come into contact with a sharlaman include:

- Does their spiritual worldview involve external entities or forces that you have to be afraid of or worship?

- Does this person act like a savior, or do they encourage you to face yourself?

- Do they ask you to become dependent on their wisdom and knowledge, or are they more interested in acquainting you with your own potential?

- Are they pointing to both your potential and the blind spots that block that potential, or are they just making you feel special?

- Is it only about exotic rituals or fancy explanations?
- How relevant are the practices and teachings to your immediate life experience?

Please answer these questions with diligence and honesty, as you may be questioning current interactions with "teachers," which is an important part of this process. Connect with your heart, which is your most important compass for assessing integrity—your own and that of a spiritual guide.

REFLECTIONS

- As Don Sinchi shared with me, hating the so-called monsters only turns you into another monster. It wasn't until I opened my heart to the disturbing experience during the second Ayahuasca ceremony that the shackles of my mind were freed, allowing Nature to embrace my entire being. *Have there been times when Nature's presence became a saving grace during a particularly difficult phase in your life? Have you had moments when you were able to feel the all-embracing and loving presence of Mother Nature, instead of identifying with the misery you may have been experiencing?*

- Don Sinchi shared that many of us have sacrificed the freedom of our aliveness in exchange for a comfortable yet numbing existence—all out of fear. *In what ways might you be willing to relinquish the fears that keep you stuck in a state of "security" so that you can experience the healing power of Mother Nature's unconditional love? What are the tangible fears you are willing to surrender to her?*

- Don Sinchi emphasized the importance of cleaning up after ourselves, both physically and energetically, to make room for evolutionary insights to integrate within us. *Are there any aspects of your life that could use some cleaning up? How can you commit to this today?*

- Don Sinchi told me that no tradition in the world has a monopoly on truth because the truth is an unconditional state of being—and moreover, the only absolute truth is that there is no absolute truth. *Do you believe this? If you do, why? And, if not, why not?*

- As Don Sinchi demonstrated in his categorization of the various types of sorcerers in Amazonian society, there is no honor in displaying empty powers without the highest integrity. Accessing the powers of Mother Nature means assuming a great responsibility, but for too many people, the demands of living in modern society can exact a toll that disempowers evolution; others often end up using spirituality for self-inflation and to perpetuate a consumerist mindset. *Have you met people who either burned out or exploited spiritual wisdom for fame, riches, and instant gratification? Have you ever been tempted to do the same?*

CHAPTER 6

THE THIRD CEREMONY

Nature Personified

After my second ceremony, so many problems and fears I hadn't been aware of had surfaced that I felt apprehensive about embarking on another ceremony so soon. However, Don Sinchi's wisdom had already earned my deepest trust and respect. With the elder's guidance, I was determined to continue, despite my inhibitions and weariness.

The ceremony started out surprisingly easy, without much physical discomfort. Don Sinchi conjured up the protective circle, and soon, my entire being was saturated with life-affirming vibrations. I initially sensed physical tremors, accompanied by vivid visions of rainforest foliage spread in fantastical designs across the earth.

Suddenly, both my physical and visionary experiences merged. I no longer had a sense of having a body; instead, I felt myself as a shimmering presence, as if I were Mother Nature personified. Mother Nature saturated what I used to call "my body" through and through. I realized that my organism was hers all along, merely entrusted into my conscious care. I found myself entirely at her mercy. She continued to arise before my inner eye:

a divine embodiment of fierce feminine love, radiating incandescent light throughout every cell.

I saw her sitting on a magnificent throne made from interwoven Ayahuasca vines decorated with brilliant turquoise leaves. Rainbow snakes coiled around her hands and legs, while her mouth opened wide in a silent roar. Her wrathful eyes pierced me. She was a pillar of love who had zero pity. I felt the Goddess of Nature expressing her trust in all her children, encouraging each of us to make it through the dark night of the soul by bowing to the divine wisdom of the heart.

Mesmerized, I surrendered. Time ceased to exist. The vibration in my being, emanating from her, became so powerful that it felt like liquefied rocks were streaming through my forehead, dense and fluid all at once. I prepared to purge. Struggling to find my way out of the maloka in the dark, I unsuccessfully tried to find the door handle for a while. The purge was already in my mouth, ready to come out, when I finally found the door. I was grateful for not purging on the maloka floor, something Don Sinchi didn't tolerate with those who'd done more than one ceremony with him.

After a tremendous purge, intense vibrations continued shaking my body; my hands, legs, and the rest of me were rhythmically vibrating. Don Sinchi came out of the maloka at a certain point to see how I was. He blew mapacho smoke at me, smiled, and said not to worry because it would pass soon. I shook a while longer and, after some time, began to feel calmer. The vibrations didn't disappear but seemed to melt into deeper, subtler levels of my being, allowing me to eventually venture back into the maloka and find my spot in the healing circle.

I continued to sit, keeping my eyes open for a while in the pitch blackness to steady my awareness. Then, Don Sinchi lit his pipe across the room from where I was sitting. The brightness of the fire from his pipe was so overwhelming that I shut my eyes. In that moment, a switch at the base of my skull turned on, enabling me to see all the people in the room as clear as daylight, with my eyes closed. I could also clearly distinguish colorful swirls of life energy traveling from the elder, clockwise in a circle, through all the participants, healing them and occasionally making some purge.

Bright filaments of light swirled through everyone in our sacred circle. I was in awe of the ceremonial space, seeing it now with my newfound faculties. That experience continued for a while before another urge to purge came. Upon returning to the maloka after my purge, my perception alternated between ordinary and energetic. My newfound sense organ located in the back of my head continued to pulsate, allowing me to perceive life energy directly. The experience lasted until the icaro that completed the ceremony and opened the magical circle was sung.

It was morning by the time we finished. The participants and Don Sinchi's apprentices had either left or fallen asleep on the floor of the maloka. Once Don Sinchi and I were the only ones left awake, he motioned me to follow him into the rainforest. I got up and found myself barely able to walk, struggling with coordination after such an intense experience. Don Sinchi, observing my challenges with understanding, let me know with his entire demeanor that it was not out of the ordinary to feel the way I felt.

Together, we walked to his favorite place at the bend of the creek.

"The third ceremony for many people is the initiation threshold," he said to me, a pleased expression on his face. "That's when people become purified enough to consciously glimpse the potential of Mother Nature's embrace. From this point on, it's possible to receive increasingly stronger glimpses of her magnificence and the potential that she represents within you."

I described to Don Sinchi my vision of the Goddess and my newfound ability to see in the dark. The elder perked up at my report, but told me not to dwell on it too much with my intellectual mind and to instead allow the extrasensory gifts to sprout within me in due time. He elaborated: "Do not be concerned with your current inability to move, because your body is still learning how to process a much greater influx of information and your newly acquired way of seeing the world. Make sure you get plenty of rest after what happened and don't get overexcited, since that would prevent miracles from becoming the new norm in your life."

Don Sinchi then accompanied me to my hut, telling me that even though I found it challenging to walk, it was necessary to integrate this new state of being into my everyday life. He recommended that after I wake up, I should walk the trails near my hut for a few hours.

Mother Nature: Embodying Eternity

I had a revitalizing rest and continued feeling the harmonizing effects of the medicine working within me. Somehow, I had a paradoxical sense of being very illuminated and yet full of questions at the same time. I went to find Don Sinchi in the hope that he could give me some answers to the questions racing inside my head. Approaching the elder's house, I saw Chispa some distance away cutting firewood; I asked him about Don Sinchi's whereabouts. Chispa was happy to see me and directed me to the chief's *chakra* ("food garden" in Kichwa).

I frantically ran in the direction Chispa pointed me to, eager to speak with Don Sinchi. More than ever, I sensed the reality of Mother Nature's organic intelligence. I was in awe of her astounding ability to communicate through the myriad life-forms in the universe, including my own body.

I found Don Sinchi in his chakra, gathering plantains. He seemed to be in a great mood, greeting me cheerfully and inviting me to give him a hand. I began helping him arrange the stacks of plantains on the ground. Before I could say anything about my experience, he observed, "You are beginning to see that she can sometimes appear in a very real way to those who are to her liking. That is very good, very good."

I begged him to tell me more about how I could establish a deeper relationship with Mother Nature.

Don Sinchi chuckled. "That is not what I was referring to when I said that she can be very real. Although she can manifest in a form recognizable to the human eye, it's still just a symbol. In reality, she is a pure force imbued with infinite, loving intelligence."

As we collected plantains, Don Sinchi invited me to sit down and enjoy the shade of the fruit trees while he shared another tale from the time of the ancestors. The Indigenous people of the Amazon had lived here, immersed in a rainforest for thousands of years. Although Nature extends to great distances in all directions, the ancestors saw it as one cohesive organism, fully conscious in and of itself. The elders of the past identified themselves and all the billions of life-forms in the rainforest as interwoven facets of the same organism. More so, they acknowledged Nature to be their greatest teacher and a symbol of higher intelligence in the universe.

"What I mean when I say that you are to her liking is not based on personal affection, but relates to emotional maturity and the cultivation of essential human qualities that are reflected energetically on the level of your being," he explained. "Without the guidance of the lineage, it's very hard, if not impossible, to see it in oneself initially. Evolution can happen only through collaboration and relatedness. Without these cornerstones, objectivity to know your highest potential can't arise."

Don Sinchi explained that the rainforest is not an easy environment to live in, given the scarcity of edible food, as well as dangerous animals, poisonous critters, and scores of other challenges. The early people who lived here did not survive in such an environment because they were stronger than it. On the contrary, they saw Mother Nature as a role model to learn from and evolve alongside. She allowed the inhabitants to thrive. Don Sinchi's ancestors recognized themselves to be an integral part of Mother Nature, alongside the rest of creation.

"People here used to live in harmony with Nature and each other, referring to the forest as Sacha Mama, which means 'Mother Forest' in Kichwa," he said. "Do you know what the first Europeans who came to the rainforest named it?! The green hell! They had that impression because of their disconnect from Nature. Being external elements in a foreign environment of the natural world reflects the state of our modern society as a whole. People are at odds with Nature and her intelligence.

"The ancient rainforest people, on the other hand, acknowledged the Spirit of Nature as the only constant in the continuous fluctuation of life and death. They witnessed the dynamic vegetation rising and falling, animals being born and dying, and all life-forms, including themselves, to be temporary occurrences within the eternal hum of the universe.

"While the ancestors discovered change to be the only constant, their greatest realization was that this change is not random at all. The cycle of life is eternally fueled by Universal Consciousness. That brilliant space you experience in ceremonies is the presence of the divine within all beings, which has never been born and will never die. The ancestors described it as the divine union of the Great Spirit's undying awareness with the Cosmic Mother's unconditional love. The direct experience of this became our people's greatest teacher of life-giving, infinite creative potential."

I interjected, telling him that my mind still struggled to see all the diverse beings as one conscious entity.

He smiled patiently. "The rainforest may initially be perceived as a combination of separate entities. However, if you look deep enough under the surface, you can see the interwoven network of tree roots, as well as the symbiotic relationships among all life-forms. The forest is also interconnected through the mycelial web. The mushroom spirits are the little helper gnomes that link the greater whole together for the messages of the unified organism to come through. When a fire rages in one part of the forest, the trees that are many days of travel away know about it almost instantaneously, thanks to the little mushroom gnomes. The trees can then fill up with more water and be less likely to be burned. Trees protect not only themselves but also many other beings in the vicinity. Everything and everyone in this environment is in sync, and every little facet supports the greater well-being of the whole organism."

He pointed to a nearby tree of delicious nuts. "There is a particular type of bee—it's the only one that can cross-pollinate the Castaña tree (Brazil nut). The shell of Castaña nuts is so strong that only one species of squirrel in the whole rainforest can crack that nut open. Then, there's only one type of fungus that can help the nuts sprout by fermenting them. Only when all those diverse life-forms come together will the Castaña tree grow, in turn supporting them all. Now, which of these beings is most important—the squirrel, the tree, the fungus, or the bee?! How about sunlight, soil, water, and air in addition to that?"

The elder, noticing that I appeared baffled by his question, answered it himself: "The Great Spirit of Unity in Diversity is what allows all of life to exist! No one can exist without everyone and everything."

After giving me a moment to take that in, Don Sinchi continued: "Similarly, within a human organism, there are many organs, systems, and cells, which initially may seem distinct and separate from each other. Yet, they all play an essential part in the human organism, which you experience in a unified way as 'yourself.' What allows the human organism to be unified is the intangible spirit of Mother Nature, which is more real than anything else. The brilliant light of consciousness necessary to see the interconnectedness of all phenomena is the Great Universal Father. The evolutionary healing path of every individual leads toward embodying the spirit of Mother Nature. We are all here to experience the divine union between the light of consciousness (the Father) and the heart's wisdom (the Mother). This is how we discover the boundlessness of Universal Love."

Don Sinchi explained that in his lineage, the aim was to relate to Nature in a personal way. That is, if Nature had a face, what face would it be, and what would it look like? If Nature had a personality, what qualities would it consist of?

It was this personification of Nature that had allowed the ancestors to attribute human qualities to the life all around them and merge the inner universe with the outer one. This allowed them to cease being intimidated by the death of their mortal shell. They realized their immortality by recognizing themselves in all beings and all beings in themselves. Without the fear of dying, their highest potential was naturally realized, because it was humbly shared in joyful service with the greater whole.

"When we share our innate gifts with each other, everyone benefits as a result," Don Sinchi said. "Collaboration, rather than competition, is the key to evolutionary healing. The radiant health of the Amazonian ancestors, documented by the first European explorers, was a direct result of such a lifestyle."

Tool: Developing a Relationship with
the Great Mother of All Life

What has your experience of Nature been? Have you seen Nature as something outside of yourself (which is not an uncommon perception among those of us brought up in the West)? Has she been something to extract resources from or something that enables you to occasionally enjoy a picturesque view? Are you afraid of nature, or do you feel a sense of fondness or connection to her? Do you see Mother Nature as a personification of organic intelligence, or does she feel more distant and foreign to you?

Considering your relationship to Nature, spend at least an hour (although more is recommended) in a natural environment without distractions. Observe how everything around you communicates and converges in a harmonious symphony. How do the various life-forms connect in an interdependent dance of creation? This will become more obvious to you if you make a habit of spending time in Nature. She will reveal herself to you and demonstrate that even the "lowliest" of creatures and organisms has an important place in the web of life.

I encourage you to further develop a relationship with Nature by personifying her, as Don Sinchi said the ancestors did. If Nature had a face, what face would it be, and what would it look like? If Nature had a personality, what qualities would it consist of? Allow your intuition to lead the way. Write down or draw what comes to you.

Modern vs. Archaic Perceptions

We sat there in the shade of the Rimyurá's garden, listening to Nature for a while. After a long, silent pause, he exhaled loudly. As I opened my eyes, he asked me if I had any questions about what he'd shared with me thus far.

"Don Sinchi, you recently mentioned that the sorcerers today work with different spirits as external forces, while in our Western world, we stopped seeing spirits altogether. Can you tell me why such a division occurred?"

Don Sinchi's face grew animated as he responded, "This is where we touch upon the difference between modern and archaic cognitive states. The ancestors perceived the world in a distinct way from modern society. Their technology was directed toward remembering the heart's infinite potential, while our current civilization prefers external technological progress to the awakening of the human spirit. Modern society largely ignores the heart by hiding it in the recesses of the mind. The degeneration of inner values is compensated by the constant upgrades of convenience-based technology to coax the mind into forgetting the heart. Yet, it's a mere illusion, created through trickery that bewitches people into a herd mentality and rules them through consumerism. Without remembering the wisdom of the ancestors, how far can we get with today's values?

"We can learn a lot from how people in archaic times experienced life. There are many myths and legends of our people that reflect the interconnected nature of our existence. Here in the rainforest, we have a rich mythic realm, personifying all life experiences to reflect the different vortexes of energy in the human organism. My great-great-grandfather was a legendary seer for our people, foretelling the disastrous events of his time and helping our people survive. He saw everyone and everything through their corresponding qualities, which are so essential for the metamorphosis of consciousness. He referred to such seeing as the language of the Great Spirit that can only be understood through *being.*"

I asked him to clarify what he meant by that.

He replied, "When the ancients had a profound sense of love, they perceived it in a relatable shape and form! They would see fairies, sprites, and all kinds of celestial beings. In the modern world, however, we just have a pleasurable sensation in our chest. When the ancestors experienced a lower vibrational frequency, such as anger or fear, they would see little monsters or demons running around. For the people today, it is mostly a rumble in the stomach or butterflies in the belly.

"Our legends state that to become skillful at their purpose as universal channels, the original ancestors gave symbolic appearances to all psychic forces. It was their way of being intimate with

103

life. The same awareness that's peeking through all beings, you and me included, has painted this physical realm with the colorful palette of life's diverse flavors. The feelings and emotions were known originally to our people as the vibrational forces of Goddess Nature because they are streamed through each of us. Our passions and inspirations, challenges and adversities, are those colorful spirits that weave our inner and outer universes together. Great art reflects the intricate designs of Spirit, but it takes even greater art to embody states of higher consciousness. The greatest art in the universe is the art of consciousness transformation.

"The original star people gave us Evolutionary Science so that we could remember consciousness transformation as the divine language of the Great Spirit. The concept of good versus bad energies didn't exist for our ancestors. Instead, they experienced the emotional energy as either heavy or light. Both are essential for the alchemy of love to heal the world. Ignorance and wisdom are also complementary opposites. Ignorance of not knowing any better is not bad in itself. When acknowledged with the heart, it becomes a fertile ground from which the wisdom of love can blossom. That is what the ancients perceived as Munaychi: the alchemical energy of love that we learn how to channel intentionally within our tradition. Munaychi is awakened through the cultivation of essential human virtues. The virtues in turn correspond to the vortexes of creative life energy within us. The momentum of Universal Love that propels us on our evolutionary journey is also known in our tradition as Munaychi."

Fascinated by the elder's account, I exclaimed that I was in awe of his ancestral culture. He quickly retorted that it wasn't *his* culture in the sense that he didn't make an identity out of it. He explained that culture should not be *bound* by ethnic context but *supported* by it. Otherwise, culture will end up an artifact in a museum, without practical application in the constantly changing world. The real meaning of culture was to keep the profound values of humanity alive across all nations. It meant that we must always remember to be humane—through wars, cataclysms, and pandemics, as well as during peaceful times.

"Sadly, over many generations, people on this planet have gradually forgotten that fact," Don Sinchi sighed. "Humanity is now lost in either the mystical world of externalized psychic forces or elaborate mental deceptions."

I felt I could see a direct connection in his words to the development of modern society. Without a conscious relationship with the inner processes of transformation, I'd noticed that people tend to go to extremes of either superstition or over-rationalization. In the Western world, around the Renaissance era in Europe, we'd experienced a total denial of the spirit realm, initiated by the advancement of empirical science. Most societies around the world quickly went from superstition to the other extreme, getting lost in the material realm of the senses. Cold rationalization of life's details had become the main authority in people's lives. It was no wonder so many of us were oblivious to the interconnected nature of reality!

Don Sinchi smiled sadly. "Yes, the devil is in the details, and as a result, life on this planet has been boiling in an unconscious pressure cooker ever since, on so many levels—from violence and disease to natural disasters. The spiritual heritage of the original ancestors was designed to reconnect us with the inner and outer universes. Once the mind understands enough to stop constantly trying to understand, it lets go of resistance to being. The sense perceptions then naturally tune in to the unified organic intelligence that's all around us."

Don Sinchi measured me with his eyes and began tying up the plantain racks for us to take back to his house. He said he would share more when we get to his house, adding, "When you get too philosophical, it's essential to balance the excessive mental energy with good physical exercise and a hearty meal to root yourself in the earth and not float aimlessly in the clouds!"

Munaychi and the Link to Creation

Once we'd returned to the elder's hut, I was curious to learn more about the mysterious Munaychi energy he'd mentioned earlier.

"If you get anything out of our talk today, it should be about the Munaychi energy that links each of us with the rest of creation," he said. "But first things first—we have to do something about your skinny energetic state of affairs." He laughed and threw a bunch of peeled plantains into a boiling pot to make our dieta meal.

After we ate the bland green plantains, which had been meticulously peeled and cooked, Don Sinchi asked with sparkling eyes, "Remember when you were a child and could play for hours outside without feeling hungry?"

"Yes, I do," I said, thinking of how I never wanted to leave my friends, even when my mother called me home for dinner. I definitely didn't experience that anymore, especially during these dietas!

Don Sinchi noted that, during childhood, we have a greater intuitive connection with Munaychi as a nourishing life force. As he said this, he seemed to transform into his childlike self; a playful expression took over his face and his wrinkles seemed to soften. I was startled at the transformation.

He noticed my reaction and said, "I mentioned to you before that we are all children of the universe, no matter how old we become. Munaychi is the energy of love that keeps us all alive, with the most essential nourishment for the soul, which resides in the heart. Without Munaychi, we would be dead on the spot. It is not some kind of mystical and mysterious energy out there that so many people tend to see it as. It is the energy of our feelings and emotions, our states of being and experiences. I can go as far as calling it the energy of each moment.

"As children, we dance with this energy without holding back and are parented by each new moment that is unlike any other that came before it. When we become 'adults,' we lose the fresh and spontaneous beginner's mind. It is the tender innocence that is so nourishing for children. We develop rigid patterns: likes, dislikes, and all kinds of personal preferences. Some moments we like and many others, we'd rather eat a cookie, which makes us childish but not childlike . . .

"For the ancestors, all of life was energy. If you resist life experience, then the same life that's meant to nurture you will exhaust you through your own resistance. It's the same energy of love—Munaychi—that can either create or destroy. Everyone serves their unique purpose within the sacred circle of life. From the womb of the Great Mother, life perpetually spirals toward the light of evolution: the Great Father. Consciously or not, we are all connected to the Great Spirit of Reciprocity, because we are all integral facets of it. For the ancestors, consciousness meant creation, and unconsciousness meant destruction. When each moment is engaged consciously from the heart, there's always a creative solution to life's predicaments. Lack of heart-centeredness, however, is a recipe for disaster. It's in such times that we struggle with the raw and uncontainable force of Nature. But after the volcano erupts, vegetation regenerates to be more resilient, lush, and vibrant than ever before. What we think of as disaster is not 'bad,' but a part of the cycle of life experience and how we access Munaychi."

Don Sinchi noticed that I was becoming overwhelmed with all this information and said, "That's enough talking for today. Take time to integrate all the lessons I am sharing with you, but don't intellectualize too much. Try to apply your ingenuity and learn how to dance with each moment, while being totally at ease. Now, go and be with yourself until you hear from me again."

Tool: Cultivating Munaychi

For many of us, learning how to be the channel, messenger, and content of the Munaychi love force, all at once, can feel both daunting and inspiring. As you consider the meaning of Munaychi—the energy of love that can either create or destroy—consider how it flows through you. Reflect on the following:

- How much of your life experience do you actually let in, moment by moment?

- Has your capacity to be tender and innocent with yourself and others changed from childhood to adulthood? How?

- How do you resist Munaychi? Notice when you tend to close down and guard your heart around some people and situations, and open up toward others. Or you may notice your resistance in your treatment of emotions. How many of them do you judge, label, repress, or cling to? If you push something away, you don't allow it to nourish you. If you cling to something or get carried away by it, you similarly prevent the energy of Munaychi from flowing through you.

- Do you tend to get lost in appearances and identities? This is another way of preventing the cultivation of Munaychi. To go beyond them, consider the part of you that experiences the world through your senses and is deeply alive. Where does it end and where does it begin? Try to find it.

REFLECTIONS

- My third Ayahuasca ceremony helped me detach from the idea of "myself," and recognize that what I thought of as me (my body, my sensations, my thoughts, etc.) was simply an instrument for the loving intelligence of the Great Mother. *Have you ever felt a time when your body wasn't your own, but an extension of nature?*

- As Don Sinchi shared with me, "Evolution can happen only through collaboration and relatedness. Without these cornerstones, objectivity cannot arise for you to know your highest potential." *Do you have any trusted wise friends on whom you can depend to be absolutely honest with you? How has this served your transformative potential?*

- The Amazonian ancestors were able to attribute "human" qualities to all of life around them because they acknowledged Nature to be an expression of infinite aliveness. This ability is what allowed them to connect their inner and outer universes—to realize that they were not separate. Moreover, it helped them recognize their own immortality, because they could see themselves in all beings and all beings in themselves. *How does fear of mortality and separation from others hold you back from realizing your highest potential in service to the greater whole?*

- Don Sinchi shared with me that he did not see his ancestral culture as belonging to him, in the sense that he didn't make an identity out of it. While cultural context is important, it can also keep us from expanding our connection to all that is. *What have you made an identity out of (sex, race, ethnicity, nationality, political ideology, etc.)? How do these aspects serve you? How might they be holding you back?*

PART 1 REFLECTION

The inner work I did with Don Sinchi influenced a deep transformation in my capacity to trust and open up to the experiential journey without letting my logical mind take over. *Move through your experiences so far, especially with the tools and reflection questions in Part 1. Have you noticed any shifts, either subtle or overt, in your own perspectives and behaviors? Have there been any challenges, small or significant? Do not be discouraged if you have encountered obstacles along the path; this is normal, and obstacles can serve to fuel your motivation rather than deter you from spiritual growth. Make a conscious commitment to awaken your heart's wisdom, and keep going!*

PART 2

DEEPENING INTO THE INDIGENOUS WORLDVIEW

CHAPTER 7

BEING WELCOMED INTO THE TRIBE

A few days after completing the three ceremonies, Don Sinchi told me: "You are now past the introductory initiation into the Evolutionary Science tradition. The next step would be to welcome you into our tribe. Throughout your healing process, you'll mostly interact with me and my immediate family. However, I will still introduce you to my people. Since you are living at my place, you are a guest of all of my tribe."

The rest of the Yahua people lived on the riverbank, about an hour away from Don Sinchi's healing center, where I'd initially arrived with my friend Sacha—a time that felt like very long ago, although it had only been a matter of weeks.

On the way there, I asked Don Sinchi why he lived so far from the rest of his people. He began by explaining that the tribe lived as one organism, with the different tasks distributed equally among everyone—just like one human being utilizes hands, legs, and the rest of the body for different purposes. Each part of our being is equally essential for the optimal functioning of the greater whole.

Don Sinchi said, "My role as a chief and a healer is similar to that of consciousness inside the organism—it's present in the body, but isn't bound by it. As a chief, I'm responsible for the well-being of our tribe so that we can be of benefit to the world around us. The chief's role is one of individuality within many tribes—often appearing quite differently from everyone else, acting unpredictably, and breaking the taboos that the rest of the tribe fears. It's done in that manner because, as a symbol of consciousness, the chief must cultivate maturity to bring fearless clarity and objectivity into every facet of tribal life."

After walking a while longer, a turn on the forest trail opened into a clearing and we entered the village. It consisted of a big field with a maloka in the middle, surrounded by traditional huts with roofs made of palm leaves. We headed toward the big communal maloka, which was three times the size of the maloka at Don Sinchi's center. Upon approaching it, I heard strange sounds, accompanied by loud breathing, coming from the inside. As we entered the maloka, I saw men and women of the tribe, young and old alike, jumping up and down in a synchronized manner, while breathing heavily and making grunting noises. Occasionally, some people were also wailing and even singing.

I asked Don Sinchi what they were doing, and he explained that this was a special energy purification practice—when the time was right, he would introduce me to it. Don Sinchi then made a loud sound, similar to a bird I'd once heard in the rainforest—it sounded like "A-yay-ma-ma!" which was also its name. Suddenly, everyone stopped and dropped to the ground. After a few minutes, people began to get up and gather around us, talking and giggling among themselves in the Yahua language.

Don Sinchi responded to them, also in the Yahua language, while pointing at me and making loud remarks. He then turned to me and explained, "There's an Amazonian fairy tale of Ayay Mama, about two children who got lost in the rainforest. After many days of wandering, they realize it is no longer possible to find their way back to their family home. With their spirit's deep longing, they magically transform into Ayay Mama birds who make the sounds of a human child calling their mama. Because they longed for motherly love so deeply, their call aids them in returning to the essence of the Great Mother. This story encourages a remembrance that we are all children of the universe, finding our way home with the bird's-eye view of our ancestors. Now that you went through the initiatory Ayahuasca ceremonies, our Yahua family can welcome you to our Sacha Mama's home."

The elder smiled, adding, "But only after you go through a special rite of passage that requires you to swim in the river."

The Yahua chief and his people all gazed curiously at me, anticipating my response. I answered that I would gladly do it, and he translated the answer to the rest of the tribe. Everyone began cheering, chanting the sound of Ayay Mama. We then proceeded in a big crowd toward the river and stopped on the sandy beach, where I undressed, jumped in the river, and swam a bit. All the Yahua people stood on the beach, laughing and screaming something incomprehensible to me. Don Sinchi then said loudly that it was the reproductive season for the piranha, and I was very brave for swimming there. Upon hearing that, I flew out of the river like a bat out of hell, making the whole tribe literally roll on the ground with laughter for several minutes. Don Sinchi, however, continued to keep a calm disposition and a polite smile.

When I approached him, he told me that I did very well and that his people would surely welcome me into their midst. Of course, I was visibly upset that he hadn't told me about the piranhas earlier!

Don Sinchi responded to me with the same polite, untroubled smile. "Although there really *are* piranhas in this river, only women with a heavy menstrual period are at risk. The tribe was just making sure you have a sense of humor, because it's an indispensable quality for our people. For us, humor is not about the ability to tell a joke. It's the ability to *take* a joke that matters." The elder looked mischievously at me.

I tried to force a smile in response, which made everyone crack up even more.

"Now, you definitely proved yourself," he said. "Welcome to the Yahuas! Now, let's go back to the village and complete the initiation!"

The Consciousness of the Tribe

Once everyone gathered in the big maloka, Don Sinchi approached a big hollow log hanging from the ceiling by sturdy ropes—it turned out to be a drum. He had a similar, smaller drum next to his maloka that he'd made by burning its core. The elder then began beating the log with a special mallet. As the drumbeat reverberated throughout the building, Chispa joined in with his flute, and everyone began dancing to the melodies in a peculiar sequence.

I was observing the celebration from outside the circle when an elderly woman came over and took me by my hand. She then hurled me into the swirling vortex of dance. After some time, I experienced a sense of lightness, while my need to maintain an image and make an impression dissolved. I could no longer sense any separation from everyone else and began to experience an exhilarating combination of presence and joy. I even joined an occasional collective yelp now and then.

After about an hour, everyone completed the dance with a synchronized primal scream, and Don Sinchi said something in Yahua to me and the old woman holding my hand. The whole tribe exploded in laughter. Suspicious, I asked Don Sinchi what he'd said.

"You see, Romancito, according to our Yahua custom, when a man accepts the invitation of a woman to join the tribal dance, they automatically become husband and wife. You can now begin a new tribal life together as a couple, never to be separated again."

I glanced briefly at the old woman, as she stared intensely back at me with a wide, toothless smile. I instantly recoiled, trying to free my hand from hers. She had an extraordinarily strong grip. Watching our struggle, Don Sinchi was no longer able to contain himself. Between fits of uproarious laughter, he tried to communicate to me, alternating words with sign language to share that everyone was just having a good joke at my expense.

After some time, everyone settled down. Don Sinchi then pulled out a ceramic vessel with black liquid from one of the shelves on the wall and came over to me with it.

"Should I drink that, Don Sinchi?"

"No, Romancito, it's not for drinking. This is *huito*, a sap from a fruit that our tribe has used since ancient times to initiate people into certain rites of passage."

The elder carefully placed his finger inside the container and painted my forehead, nose, cheeks, hands, and legs with the black liquid. He then pulled out a mirror from another shelf and showed me my reflection; the marks on my cheeks resembled cat whiskers. Don Sinchi explained that the legends mentioned that the Yahua people's ancestors were able to shape-shift, and their favorite form was that of a big, wild cat.

"As we receive you into the Yahua nation, we also welcome you to our cat family—*Michi Ayllu* in Kichwa," he explained.

As the tribal dancing, celebration, and chatter went on throughout the initiation, Don Sinchi took me by my hand and whispered in my ear, "Come now, it's time for us to get back to the healing center before our people make more fun of you."

Don Sinchi then made a roar that resembled that of a jaguar, and everyone started coming to us, one by one, embracing both me and the Rimyurá to bid us farewell. On the way back through the forest, we sat on an old fallen log for a moment. The sunset was just beginning, with gentle rays of shimmering colors streaming through the many layers of the leaves above us.

Although I was enjoying the peace of this moment, in such contrast to the raucous tribal welcoming ceremony, I also wished to understand more about the Yahua culture.

I said, "Don Sinchi, you mentioned today on our way to the village that you are the consciousness of the tribe. Why doesn't everyone in the tribe cultivate their own consciousness?"

The Yahua chief replied, "In the old days, it was that way—every member of the tribe was the chief, equally responsible for themselves and everyone else. Everyone cultivated their consciousness to its highest potential while maintaining cooperation, love, and harmony with each other. Our Yahua people loved the spacious freedom that higher consciousness brings. In ancient times, our tribe was not as you saw it today, with houses so close to each other. Each family lived at least half a day's walk from each other, and yet, somehow, everyone knew what everyone else in the tribe was up to. Each family was fully responsible for stewarding the rainforest half a day's walk in each direction.

"Because our people lived so spaciously, the conquistadors didn't capture us so easily. Our freedom also protected us from the smallpox pandemic and weakened the ability of the missionaries to indoctrinate us. However, over time, our people gradually succumbed to the ignorance of egocentric behavior. Once the forgetfulness set in, people became divided and fearful, needing leaders who exemplified the primordial wisdom of interconnectedness. My job is to keep conjuring the most optimal strategies for keeping my people and our ancestral wisdom alive, alongside my healer friends across the Amazon basin."

Out of adaptation to the rapidly changing times, the elders of previous generations had implemented the way of life I'd been introduced to today. Don Sinchi's people survived by keeping the evolutionary wisdom alive in at least a few among the many of them. The Rimyurá was the one who had a responsibility to guide people through the dream of separation in both the physical and spiritual realms.

"My main responsibility is to listen and observe before responding," Don Sinchi said. "I make sure that my people are truly well in their hearts and have an abundance of love in their lives. Not everyone in the tribe wants to know about the intricacies of higher consciousness. In fact, most of our people today are satisfied with the idea that the chief and the council of elders take care of that."

The elder looked attentively at me and asked if, in my Western culture, we had ways of taking young people through rites of passage that would help them mark the stages of their evolution. I thought about it and said, "In the West, we have educational institutions, where children get the necessary foundation for adult life."

Don Sinchi smiled. "Yes, your world teaches all kinds of topics, except the most essential one: how to live life to the fullest, all while bringing the greatest benefit to everyone around! For my people, on the other hand, this is the most essential curriculum. Our heritage was destined to help bring profound human values back into the world and restore the original meaning of the word *culture* to society."

"Do you think human civilization is not evolving, Don Sinchi?"

"It's evolving, just not in a very conscious, voluntary, or harmonious way. In mainstream society today, the primary focus is on material values. A heart-centered transformation of consciousness is not honored in a world ruled by greed. The staggering number of wars, natural disasters, sicknesses, and diseases, as well as the degree of poverty and famine in the world, all reflect the currently distorted values of humanity. The degradation of human values, through overconsumption and separation, leads to decay. For evolutionary healing to sweep our planet, uniting our diversity is essential."

I remembered the 9/11 terrorist act, which had occurred within two weeks of my arrival in the Amazon for the very first time. Sad and terrible as it was, my friends in New York had shared with me that the event completely changed the way people related to one another afterward. New York was famous for the rude behavior of its people, but the collective tragedy had united New Yorkers as a community. Facing a common threat had ushered them into an evolutionary state, and they'd become compassionate and considerate of each other.

Don Sinchi said, "In ancient times, people figured out a way to face their shadows voluntarily and consciously, thus preventing or minimizing the possibility of getting hurt. By not reconciling the issues directly, our shadows are projected externally, causing harm to others and to ourselves, which only perpetuates collective suffering. Have you ever noticed how in war, the other side is always demonized? I have seen some wars in my life, living close to the borders of Peru, Colombia, Brazil, and Ecuador. All wars, dis-eases, and calamities on Earth are the result of unresolved inner conflicts on a mass scale. Such was the observation of the enlightened ancestors. I completely agree with them through my experience!"

Tool: Coming Together

Who are the people in your life that are part of your intentional community? These are not necessarily the people who have the same belief system as you, but people with whom you don't have to pretend or keep up appearances—you can just be yourself. These are the ones with whom you can get real and who will encourage you in the midst of struggle—and vice versa. These are also the ones with whom you can easily share your well-being. Write down a list of all the people you've considered to be a part of your beloved community, as well as the qualities of your connection. Even if you only write down the names of a couple people, the kind of community to cultivate is about quality rather than quantity. Next, write down a list of all the actions you're willing to take to ensure that you can gather with beloved community, intentionally and steadily.

Awakening to the Initiation

At this stage of my time in the Amazon, I was curious as to how I could verify the wisdom of the ancients by applying it more directly to my own experience. I had thus far heard many profound teachings, but aside from the three ceremonies, how could I embody these teachings more continuously?

The elder thought about it before replying, "The three ceremonies you recently experienced together were a rite of passage, aiming to return you to your true nature by helping you take full responsibility for your life. You do so by recognizing the value of your life in relation to life all around you. Here, you go through a similar rite of passage as the people of New York, but consciously and voluntarily. You are being guided by the living wisdom of the ancestors in a safe, intentional, supportive space."

The Rimyurá paused, and I saw kindness glistening in the deep pools of his eyes. After a prolonged moment, he invited me to ask a question. I decided to ask something that had troubled me ever since Don Sinchi had shared the demise of his people.

"So, if the Amazonian people had gone through their rites of passage consciously and voluntarily, the cataclysmic event where most of the Indigenous Amazonians perished in the fifteenth century wouldn't have happened?"

His expression changed into grave concern. "Yes, sadly, as I shared with you before, during that time, a lot of confusion and separation had already taken over most of our people's minds. It was the end of a glorious era for the Amazonian kingdom, which was founded by enlightened ancestors. The cataclysm in this part of the world was a result of mass amnesia. The only people to survive were the ones who recognized what was happening as an unconscious ceremony. It was a big wake-up call for our people. Many did not heed it, all the way to the bitter end.

"Those who survived did so through their ability to see the essence beneath appearances. The ancient seers understood how the pandemic of forgetfulness works, and because of that, they could also foresee the future. They then organized the living lineages to carry distinct aspects of Evolutionary Science through the generations, all the way to this time, so that we would be able to remember ourselves. The Yahuas were among the first who had direct contact with the first European explorers, and yet, we have survived, while many other tribes perished. Our elders say it's because our tribe unites several of those ancient lineages that were left for us to caretake by the original ancestors. We do so not just for our own sake, but because this path is a saving grace for all of humanity."

"And the initiation I have received today, Don Sinchi?" I inquired.

"What you experienced when our people were making fun of you was a cleansing rite to welcome you into our tribe. The Yahua heritage is to be free people. You must loosen up and not take yourself too seriously if you are to become a free human being!"

Noticing how I was reflecting on getting upset at the different jokes played on me at various points throughout the day, the elder stopped talking and grinned at me. Gradually, a reddish glow began to reflect the darker hues of the vegetation around us, and the insects initiated their moonlight orchestra. Without much daylight left, we got up and proceeded back to Don Sinchi's center.

As we approached my hut, the elder looked at me with a kind smile, nodded toward the hut, and left me to be with myself. Alone now, I continued to reflect on the interconnected alliance of enlightened ancestors working across time and space to continue guiding humanity. These thoughts brought me great inspiration, allowing me to rest and not feel so lonely in the modern world.

Tool: Connecting with the Enlightened Ancestors

You may wish to create your own rite of initiation into a new, more intentional phase of your life. A simple but effective way, whether just with yourself or with friends, is to meditate with a small, naturally made drum. In the Amazonian tradition, the drum represents the first sound we hear in our mother's womb—her heartbeat—which is why it was used in the tribal welcoming ceremony. Flutes, shakers, and other tribal instruments may also be used.

Create a meditative rhythm that is synchronized with your breath. Close your eyes. Next, visualize your ancestral and current tribe all around you, welcoming you on your journey; humbly ask them to guide you. Then, let go of all thoughts and be fully present with your breath and the drumbeat. Journal after the practice if particular shapes, animals, or people emerged in your visions. What are the defining qualities of your visions? What feelings do they evoke in you?

Practice for at least 20 to 30 minutes at a time, two or three times a week, for a deeper connection.

REFLECTIONS

- Don Sinchi shared with me that, even in times of darkness and global confusion, the wisdom of the ancestors continues to accompany us all. The ancestors could foresee the hurdles of a gradually increasing planetary crisis. *In what ways have you relied on ancient wisdom to help you meet the times we find ourselves in?*

- To ward off the pandemic of forgetfulness, Don Sinchi's living wisdom lineage requires that each member in the tribe go through at least the most basic rites of passage of facing oneself. The Yahua mystery school offers initiations that delineate the foundational stages of each individual's evolution. Everyone is also provided with a clear glimpse of more advanced stages, should they choose to pursue them. *What has your experience of initiation been in the culture in which you live? What might be missing in the rites of passage you are familiar with?*

- Don Sinchi told me that all the disasters and cataclysmic events that occur regularly nowadays are wake-up calls, encouraging everyone to remember why we're here. Instead of heeding the urgent sounds of the apocalyptic alarm clock, however, humanity keeps hitting the snooze button. Modern society continues to invite more cataclysms to shake us out of a collective slumber. As a whole, we unconsciously long for the collective awakening of the heart, but we individually fear facing our shadows. To be sustainable, evolution must be conscious and intentional. *How, in your life, are you walking a path of evolution— not just for yourself but also for global consciousness?*

- I learned from Don Sinchi time and again that the ego loves the leading role in the drama of life. This is why a sense of humor is essential when it comes to snapping out of the drama and remaining in our hearts. Don Sinchi shared that a good sense of humor is more about how you take a joke rather than tell one. Once you know who you truly are, there'll be nothing anyone can ever say or do to upset you. *What's your sense of humor like? How good are you at taking a joke? How can this be an important spiritual lesson for your ego?*

- In the beginning of the dark ages, there were enlightened beings who stayed behind in different parts of the world to help guide humanity through the darker times. The intergenerational lineages of uninterrupted living wisdom were born in power centers across the planet. Each of these traditions maintains a connection with the same enlightened stream of primordial consciousness as the people of the Amazon, but from a different angle. Each lineage expresses the same essence with a unique style that's relevant to a distinct cultural context. *What wisdom traditions have captured your heart over the years? How have they taught you to enter into the Evolutionary Science you've learned about by reading this book?*

CHAPTER 8

THE WAVE OF REMEMBRANCE

After that introduction to the rest of the Yahua tribe, many days of solitary stay in my dieta hut ensued. It was the rainy season, so torrential downpours had flooded large portions of the rainforest around us. At times, it seemed like buckets of water were pouring from the clouds for days on end. The once-modest creek next to Don Sinchi's house turned into a small river carrying huge trunks of trees brought down by lightning. It was a suitable time for introspection, and I was able to reflect more clearly on the healing journey I'd found myself so deeply immersed in.

One day, Don Sinchi struck up a conversation by asking me how I was doing.

"I am incredibly grateful to you, Don Sinchi," I said. "The last Ayahuasca ceremony we had together, where I was able to see with my eyes closed, dissolved whatever doubts were still lingering about your tradition. A humming sensation in the back of my head, accompanying my newfound clear sight, continues to be with me, even now, as we speak. These new abilities, however, seem to be fading."

The elder measured me quietly before speaking. "The momentum of your habitual life is still strong, and because of that, your perception is slowly returning to the realm it's habituated to. The more you experience the ways of the ancients, the more your perception will be inclined to remain in the evolved paradigms of life.

Now is a good time to introduce you more deeply to our ancestral ways. Do you remember the talk we had the day we met?"

"Yes, of course. How can I forget the story of enlightened ancestors?"

"I mentioned to you at that time that Evolutionary Science was a way to merge the river of individual consciousness with the celestial ocean of divine awareness."

"Yes, I recall. It's a beautiful metaphor, Don Sinchi."

"It is far from being just a metaphor—it's an actual discipline, and it's about time to start applying it in your life!"

Don Sinchi went on to tell me that the Amazon River was called the River Ocean in ancient times. The ancestors had considered it to be the primary stream of enlightened awareness into which many spiritual tributaries merged. Each tributary represented a sacred set of instruments in Evolutionary Science. For all these diverse instruments to be applied skillfully, the Indigenous people had a series of foundational practices that were implemented either before or after the first three Ayahuasca ceremonies, depending on the predisposition of each apprentice. The purpose of these practices was to transform all inner conflicts into a healing balm for the soul.

The elder looked at me to see if I was following along. "This occurs when we bring awareness into every moment and aspect of our life. This is not an easy task, as it requires immense motivation. Just doing it for your own sake will not suffice."

He explained that the River Ocean began as a drop of water or even a snowflake, high in the Andes. On their journey down, more and more drops came together. Every drop willing to join a cause greater than its individual self made the arduous possibility of reaching the distant Ocean of the Awakened Shared Heart a reality. In the same way, the drop of our individual consciousness can join the enlightened stream of awareness, alongside multitudes of other beings from past, present, and future. This is why we must remember that we're not separate drops reaching for the ocean, but an ocean of Universal Love inside the drop of our own individual awareness.

"After all, what is an ocean if not a collection of individual drops?" Don Sinchi mused. "The ancestors saw that we are all inexorably linked to the universe around us. The separation we experience between ourselves and the rest of this vast existence is an illusion that we make real by believing in it. Just like the drops are not separate from the ocean and the trees are inseparable from the forest, where you end and others begin is a fine line. By relating to everyone in your life as unique reflections of your greater self, you reconcile your inner imbalances."

The Journey of Remembrance

Don Sinchi went on to share that the journey of remembrance necessitates the purest of intentions and undeterred striving, because you are remembering your own childlike innocence. A natural state of well-being is the essential truth of all our lives. Although this state is intuitively known to each of us since before birth, we confuse it for the circumstances that encourage us to experience it. It's like the sun that's reflected in many puddles of water—but while each puddle reminds us of the sun, none of them can provide the warmth and light that can only come from the source.

The wish to consciously realize our intuitive knowing beyond illusory appearances serves as a catalyst for the evolutionary journey. This is when the heart begins to relate with others. The wish for realizing the source of who we are may come from either not getting what we want, or getting it but not being satisfied with our conditional happiness. The momentum of countless beings, all reaching toward being loved and being able to love, can then propel us to accomplish the inconceivable—which is the boundless capacity of the heart to transcend all limitations.

Don Sinchi shared that the reason Evolutionary Science had always revolved around healing was that the enlightened ancestors' original intention was to bring humanity back into a state of interconnectedness—something he'd shared with me countless times before. Once we begin to see ourselves in others and others in ourselves, through all our struggles and successes, genuine healing becomes possible. The Great Spirit of Unconditional

Love can only be experienced fully once our consciousness is all-encompassing and all-relating. Humanity's shared heart is an indispensable support on the heroic journey toward the totality of being.

"In the old times, the healers who worked for the benefit of all beings were known as the greatest ones," he said. "To attain such mastery, you must realize that suffering is not what makes you special. The collection of all your issues brought together serves as the fertile ground for your most genuine healing to unfold from. Conscious or not, everyone is on a heroic evolutionary journey. All beings are going through the same process in their own unique way. This recognition is what allows individual identity to dissolve its illusory separation from others. The awakening of the heart's wisdom necessitates supporting everyone in our life on their journey. Seeing the Great Spirit in all beings and under all circumstances allows the seed of the heart to gestate and eventually be born from the dark womb of conditioned existence.

"Mother Nature teaches that the more you share, the more you have. As you are healing, with a motivation that is greater than yourself, you are simultaneously maturing to be of greater benefit to the world. If your goal is only to heal for your own sake, however, happiness will be short-lived. True happiness is only possible when it's shared. In the old times, people recognized each other as themselves—not in terms of you being the exact replica of me, but in the sense that we are all unique emanations of the Great Spirit. Our ancestors recognized the collective spirit of our interconnectedness to be the greatest spirit of all."

Don Sinchi's words were compelling. I liked imagining the ocean as a conscious organism of which the individual self is but a drop. In its totality, the ocean is the Great Spirit that the individual self merges with.

"Remember how unconsciousness means resistance, and consequently, decomposition?" Don Sinchi asked. "The individual drops shatter, just so they can become one with everything. But for the drop that is ignorant of that fact, the experience is so terrifying that it loses all its senses in the shattering and sinks into an oblivion of deep slumber. In reality, what gets shattered is our obsession with the idea that there's a solid, separate self called an I. By identifying with this illusion, the fragmented awareness of the drop becomes even more lost in the murky waters of ignorance. That's how we end up in this material dimension of misleading appearances and continue to have the same recurring dream of being isolated from the whole."

I knew very well what it was like to harbor the fear of my individual self being eradicated. I thought of the many stories of people who'd had great spiritual awakenings, only to fall into a psychosis or meltdown. Although they may have been on the cusp of a breakthrough, it was ultimately their resistance to merging with the greater ocean of consciousness that perpetuated a sense of terror.

"The great ocean is always communicating to the deluded drops that we are," Don Sinchi went on. "When we listen to the ocean, it helps us realize we've been a drop in the ocean all along. When we listen to our mental fabrications, we dream of separate selves, enslaved by impulses, desires, adversities, and fears. The Great Spirit teaches us to be aware, so that ultimately, we can awaken from the mother of all dreams: the illusion of separation. The first rule of thumb to dreaming awake is not to wallow in one's own misery and to keep looking further than one's own nose."

I asked, "Are you saying the dreams we are having at night are actual communications of the higher self?"

The Rimyurá smiled mischievously. "I am saying that our entire life is a wake-up call from the dream of separation. You dream at night, and during the day you are being dreamed. Yes, the dreams are actual communications, but not in the way we tend to think of communication. The Banco Muraya sorcerers say that Mother Nature talks in a very different language from human beings. It's a language that is woven from creative potential and metaphors, not dry logic. That's why you'll find so many paradoxes on the path of Evolutionary Science. The conceptual mind keeps getting entangled in the infinite mystery until it learns to get out of its own way."

"So then, how would I go about interpreting my dreams?" I asked, trying to find a practical approach to what he was saying.

"The dreaming wave practice is another tributary of Evolutionary Science we'll explore at another time. For now, I want to introduce a practice you can begin to cultivate in your waking life as an essential foundation to your spirit path. The first practice for returning to the ocean is called 'the wave of remembrance.' Your initial engagement with this wave begins by recalling all the people you've ever met in your life. You must learn to see everyone as drops, emerging from the same ocean and returning to it. Then, through love, breath, and forgiveness, you can start to dissolve any tensions involving yourself and others back into the ocean of your heart-centered presence."

He explained that our personalities are shaped by all the people we've ever met, starting with our parents. Our personality is a conduit for universal life force, which is not some kind of mystical energy that exists "out there." Rather, this life force streams through us as long as we're alive—and it's often too obvious for us to even notice. Any unresolved emotional knot in relation to a person or situation from our past distorts our ability to be a clear channel. When the natural life force doesn't flow harmoniously, physical and psychological imbalances occur.

"The sacred plants can be skillful instruments of the remembrance practice," Don Sinchi continued. "Sometimes, during a ceremony, a troublesome event from your life can emerge for you to face, accept, and transform through loving presence. You have already had a chance to do that in the three ceremonies with me so far. The purpose of our tradition, however, is for your whole life to become a ceremony. We drink Ayahuasca with the willingness to open our hearts to all of life's adversities. The commitment to getting to know all of your good, bad, and ugly parts is essential. Only through reconciliation and openheartedness toward yourself can you stop living in an elaborate self-deception and start becoming a real human being."

"So, does that mean I have to forget my past?"

"No, silly! You do not forget your past; however, you *do* release all the emotional tensions trapped in it that prevent you from experiencing life to the fullest in the here and now. On the path of returning to the ocean, there should be nothing in the past that one holds on to, for even the positive and exciting energies can be a trap. If all you do is think of how good life used to be, how can you enjoy the present?"

He stopped to think for a moment. "All those people and events in your life are messengers of the Great Spirit—the formless within the form. Some inspire you to be a real human being, and some challenge you to walk your talk. The practice of remembrance is about taking to heart all the lessons of life. Instead of trying to change or erase your past, you begin to see how your unresolved issues are still controlling your behavior in the present. Once you can remain steadfast under pressure and turmoil, you will know that you're mastering this practice."

The Anchor of Awe and Wonder

In the following rainy weeks, the wave of remembrance completely engulfed me. I stayed the entire time in my hut, consuming the plant medicines that Don Sinchi saw fit for me. When I asked him why he'd waited all that time to prescribe plants, he said that because my illness was genetic and chronic, it had many subtle energetic knots. In my case, my mind first had to open up to the idea that total healing was even possible. That could only occur once I'd begun to understand my disease as an expression of evolutionary love, a wake-up call to honor the calling of the heart.

The elder instructed me to focus on remembering my earliest childhood memories, which represented an innocent, childlike state of being. Don Sinchi elaborated that "childlike" had nothing to do with temper tantrums or immature behavior. As children, we are closer to the creative source on an intuitive level and engage life with a sense of adventure and awe toward the Great Mystery. A beginner's mind is essential to start seeing all our curses as blessings in disguise.

Initially, my mind resisted the practice, and I constantly became distracted. Don Sinchi advised, "Try to describe your memories from a third-person perspective, and then imagine how that person must've felt."

I had to put a lot of effort into transcribing the events, which at first echoed vaguely in my memory, into a notebook that Don Sinchi permitted me to keep for this task. Finally, after persevering with the slow and steady breathing that accompanied the detailed visualizations of my life events, the ice cap around my heart began to melt. I realized that my initial resistance had come from my deeply ingrained fear of being vulnerable. Once I began to face my inhibitions, they became portals into different times and places in my life. Then, one day, unexpectedly, the events of my life came flooding effortlessly into my daily awareness. I could suddenly see, smell, and hear all the details of memories all the way into early childhood. At Don Sinchi's request, I recounted to him my earliest memories when he visited my hut.

My first significant flashes of memory involved growing up in the Eastern European country of Moldova, which at that time was still a republic under the Soviet regime. For the first nine years of my life, I lived in the countryside, on the outskirts of a large town. My family's small house was built by my great-grandfather and had a relatively big front yard. It was an old, one-bedroom house with a small bathroom, which functioned simultaneously as a coal furnace and a boiler room in wintry weather. The water pipes passing through the furnace circumvented and heated the entire house in the snowy winters. The living room was wallpapered with floral designs, and a pendulum clock with ancient Roman numbers etched into it hung on the wall. The black-and-white TV set, which was rarely watched and most frequently used as a flower stand, was also an essential part of the decor.

My parents turned their bedroom into a children's nursery when I was born, and once I became a toddler, they moved their bedroom into the living room, leaving me with my own space. Recollections of an old tapestry, with intricate designs of dogs and horses, that hung over my crib brought me back to the most cherished and long-forgotten memories.

At first there was just the magical silence, accompanied by my mother's loving lullabies and her nurturing embrace. Spending many hours alone in the comforting darkness, I was fascinated by the tiny sparkling lights that my eyes could distinguish in the pitch-black screen of night. Those magical sparkles wove the fabric of reality that was just for me to experience.

Both my parents worked full time—my mother as an art teacher and my father as a mechanical engineer. The many days I spent alone were filled to the brim with enchantment. Every corner of the house was imbued with meaning and mystery. I could spend hours exploring that seemingly small yet endlessly vast universe of our residence.

When my parents were home, I could hear the muffled sound of arguments behind the walls. Although they hid their quarrels from me at first, the atmosphere was often tense, making it challenging for me to be playful and lively.

However, even within the unsettling energy of our home, I felt protected by higher forces. After my mom put me to bed at night and I lay in the room by myself, an invisible entity would lift the blanket off me, and with great care, lay it back on my body. A gentle hand would then land on my ankle, bringing me into a deep, peaceful state. I felt profoundly cared for, which allowed me to sink into a deep sleep filled with beautiful dreams.

At the age of four, when my rational mind was more coherent, I began to fear that invisible entity because I lacked a rational explanation for it. One night, as the sheets were being lifted off my body and the moonlight illuminated the room, I opened my eyes and looked up. What I saw was an outline of a tremendous furry creature looming over me—not unlike the Chewbacca character from *Star Wars*. I somehow intuitively knew that it had only the kindest and most loving intentions toward me, but my fear of what I couldn't explain caused me to scream out. My parents, who were right outside the door, instantly rushed in, just in time to witness my blanket mysteriously drop from thin air to the floor. Of course, they dismissed all of it, saying it had just been my imagination. Still, I remembered it vividly and told all my friends in kindergarten that a bear was protecting me at night.

Don Sinchi especially liked these memories and took the time to reflect on them with me.

"The Indigenous people of the Amazon say that human beings are meant to be happy. It's our original birthright and heritage.

The only thing that prevents us from experiencing timeless joy is our own forgetfulness and the ignorance of not knowing any better. The carefree memories of the inner child are your own insights into the primordial truth.

"The focus of the wave of remembrance is one's own original, natural state of well-being. You scout out the state of your true nature by tracking down your vulnerable traits, such as openness, awe, faith, kindness, tolerance, and a whole array of other essential human qualities. These glimpses were inscribed into you at different times of your life as evolutionary seeds. You can bring them to life once you're mature enough to remember your higher purpose. In the inner abode of Mother Nature, just like in the outer wilderness, you must follow the footprints of life experience to find your way home."

Tool: The Wave of Remembrance

Take some intentional time for this practice, which you'll continue to add on to with the remaining practices in this book.

Start by remembering the earliest, purest, most joyful, and innocent memories of your life. Feel the sensations these experiences elicited. This will establish an anchor of well-being as a point of reference to which you may always return. Honoring and making a discipline out of cultivating this original state will also help you see how it gets clouded by all the disturbances in your life. The motivation to embody the anchor of well-being more fully can help you steadfastly face the dynamics with people from your past with whom you still have unresolved emotional charges.

The Wild Forces of Nature

"Is the practice to cultivate the essential human qualities under all circumstances? Obviously, it's easier to do this in more encouraging circumstances, but am I to learn how to be open, kind, and tolerant . . . even when things aren't going so well?" I asked the elder.

Don Sinchi nodded and responded, "That furry creature who visited you regularly, early on in life, was your *don*. In Evolutionary Science, this is the dream body of your higher self. Your don cares for and protects the essence of Nature within you from the moment you are born. For our people, they are messengers of Goddess Nature, making sure we remember her upon 'growing up.' For different people, these messengers may appear differently, but the essence of the message will always remain the same. Even ferocious, hairy creatures have this intuitive knowledge of how unconditional love is the source of all true power in the world. Most people, due to a disconnect between rationality and intuition, either forget or dismiss those experiences of 'invisible friends' as figments of their imagination later in life."

The elder's response reminded me of another memory from when I was five or six years old. I shared with him that whenever I didn't feel in agreement with the energy at home, I'd run off to climb a big hill, located some distance away from our house. I would bring a small chair along to sit and reflect on my life from a higher perspective. Engaging the wave of remembrance, while being alone in the hut, I could see how those were my initial attempts at contemplative meditation, intuitively done in solitude, away from turmoil.

On that spot, I remembered conversing with three invisible friends whom only I could see. They began appearing in my life when I was about three years old and always showed up in times of crisis to keep me company. All of them were older men with beards, and each gave me useful advice in their own unique way. One was serious and quiet, another kind and wise, and the third humorous and chatty.

The last time I saw them was when I was nine years old and was hit by a car as I crossed the road on my bicycle. I didn't initially understand what had happened: one moment I was on the bicycle, and the next, my entire world was swirling all around me. The next thing I knew, I was on the ground, unable to get up, with many people gathered around me. Someone kept placing an ammonia inhalant under my nose so that I wouldn't lose consciousness. Then, an ambulance came and took me to the hospital. While I was in the emergency room, my three bearded friends suddenly appeared. They said this would be the last time they'd appear until a moment in the distant future. They told me not to worry and that I would be fine because God was watching over me. I wasn't raised religious and didn't understand what they meant, but for some reason, it made me relax throughout the ordeal. My friends vanished into thin air, and in the next instant, the door to my hospital quarters swung open and my mother rushed in.

I learned later that a friend saw me get hit by a car and immediately ran to our house, calling for help. When he told my mom about the accident, she asked him whether I was alive or not. His honest answer was that he didn't know. Upon hearing this, she immediately bolted out of our house to find me. She neither cared for her appearance nor about injuring her bare foot on the sharp rocks along the way (she lost one slipper while getting there). That was a powerful glimpse of just how profound her love for me was.

I was released from the hospital that day with a hematoma on my right leg and a cast. I spent most of my summer vacation that year recovering in a horizontal position in the grapevine gazebo in our front yard. My grandfather had planted it long before I was born to make his own wine since our region was known for its vineyards. I could vividly recall the ripe grapes hanging from the vines within arm's reach and the sour shoots I'd enjoyed chewing on. My grandfather was known to be a wise man in our community, and his wisdom now resonated for me with the Amazonian tradition of planting the seeds of truth.

As far as the three wise men were concerned, it was only much later in my life that I saw references to them in the tales and legends of diverse cultures around the world—particularly in the story of the birth of Jesus, which brought great tidings from three wise men from the East.

Don Sinchi commented, "You shouldn't take it too literally and expect to one day meet three older men with beards who like to hang out together! Instead, it's much more meaningful to see those three men as aspects of your higher self."

He explained that, as children, we intuit the essential qualities that are most supportive to us on life's evolutionary journey. A serious, contemplative attitude is essential for exposing superficial values. A kind, wise attitude helps us transform habits of destructive ignorance. The ability to smile at oneself in the midst of drama is instrumental, so as not to lose our spark due to everyday wear and tear.

I then shared with Don Sinchi another powerful memory that had come tumbling back into my awareness. Nomadic gypsies who had a lot of horses lived near my childhood home. From a young age, I was inexplicably drawn to horses; I saw them as majestic beings, filled with grace and power. Throughout my childhood, I often snuck out of my house to go to the pastures and feed grass to the horses for hours on end.

On one occasion, five gypsy children befriended me, and I brought them to our house for lunch. My mother always welcomed our guests with great hospitality. When they left, however, my mother discovered that they'd stolen all our shoes. I was reprimanded, and my mom made me promise never to bring them over again. A quarrel with the gypsy kids ensued shortly after, ending in us throwing rocks at each other. We fortunately missed one another by a mile, and no one was hurt.

Although I continued to feed the gypsies' horses, I avoided the children from that point on. A few months after our conflict, I fed a beautiful white stallion one day. The horse bent its head, and as I approached, it unexpectedly straightened, headbutting me in the chest. I flew several feet backward, and although I had a soft landing, it took a while to restore my knocked-out breath and get up. That experience made me fear horses for many years, until my 20th birthday, when I mustered the courage to take lessons at a horse academy. Despite my fears, my fascination with horses continued throughout my life. Even in the years when I was afraid to ride them, I drew them and thought of them constantly.

Don Sinchi commented on this memory as well. "A horse has become your power animal since that memorable event, and the spirit of the horse comes to help you in challenging situations. Remember how in the intensity of an Ayahuasca ceremony, you described the vibrations you were feeling to be akin to a racing horse? When there is a strong encounter with an animal like that, it leaves an imprint on the energy body. Consequently, whenever we encounter difficult situations, our psyche imitates the qualities of the creature that made a strong imprint in the stream of our awareness. It's an intuitive human response to danger: to act out that which you found scary in the past, in order to fend off new threats. For example, if you were scared by a jaguar in the past, you will imitate its behavior when in danger, perhaps even roaring like the animal that once caused such a fright. We Yahuas have a rite of passage in which a young warrior goes into the rainforest to face a ferocious animal. Whether he succeeds in overcoming the animal or not is irrelevant. As long as the initiate survives that encounter, the spirit of the animal becomes their guardian spirit for life."

I deeply resonated with that perspective and even remembered a poem I'd written as an ode to my kinship with horses. It was from my late teenage years—a time in my life when my interest in the natural healing path was just beginning.

The Yahua elder clapped his hands and laughingly said, "I knew there was a poet hiding in you! That's an important part of your essential humanity. The wave of remembrance is effective only when you recognize a higher wisdom in all the dynamics of your life. Your love of horses is a great example of an anchoring memory from the time in your life when you experienced the untamed nature of innocence, while also getting in trouble because of it. Despite the rational mind, which instilled fear around your primal self, the poet in you was in awe of the wild forces of nature.

"Awe is what allows the shadows in our lives to be integrated and transformed into the light of consciousness. The heart of Mother Earth's dark womb is a creative fire seed, bursting with infinite possibilities that yearn to be born into a higher conscious existence. The light of your awareness is seeded inside the shadow realm, so you can discover your even greater potential to shine more brightly."

After evaluating my state of being with his crystal-clear gaze, Don Sinchi concluded, "You have established the foundation for your purest memories; now they can be portals into your divine nature, which you can fully manifest into existence. You can now follow the timeline of your life and bookmark the moments when your innocence was wounded, and when you retreated into a protective shell."

With the original memories of childlike wonder as a point of reference, it definitely became easier for me to gain more insight; all the incidents that had distanced me from my carefree innocence were the footprints leading me back home.

Tool: Healing Your Wounded Innocence

Another name for the disease of forgetfulness, as Don Sinchi informed me, is *soul loss*. *We can engage with the process of retrieving our soul in this next step of practicing the wave of remembrance by applying the anchor of openhearted inspiration when it comes to our more difficult memories and traumas. This is how we can begin to heal our wounded innocence.*

Start with a positive memory first, to establish an anchor of well-being to cultivate through more challenging memories; this positive memory is a bookmark to which you can always refer.

As you breathe in, remember all the details of a particular memory, and as you breathe out, try to embody the state of being you experienced at the time of the event. Did your body feel at ease, restful, energized, nurtured, taken care of? The bodily experience is an essential reference point in the practice.

The next step in the practice is to write down all the key events from your childhood up until now. Pick one and go through it thoroughly before moving on to the next one. Try to go to the earliest memories, but it's also fine to engage more recent ones. *Do not focus on the most traumatic or difficult memories; we will get to these in a later chapter.* Instead, focus on the ones with a "medium" charge.

It can be helpful to begin with memories of your mother and father, because it all starts there. Be present and breathe through the memories until there is no longer an energetic charge left in them and the body no longer needs to be reminded to be at ease.

REFLECTIONS

- The Great Spirit is continuously imparting love to each of us through the interactions with all the beings in our life. As Don Sinchi shared with me, only with the ingenuity of our shared heart can we hope to embody the Great Spirit of infinite human potential. *In what ways do you hold back from recognizing your connection to all beings, including the ones who may have caused you pain? How can you begin to transform this pain into valuable lessons that help you cultivate the essential qualities of your true nature?*

- Don Sinchi continually showed me that, to reach my full potential, it was necessary to expose my self-imposed limitations. I had to apply my trust in Mother Nature in order to face the wounds of my body and soul. To rise into the light of my highest purpose, it was necessary to root deeply in love, empathy, and compassion. Yet, despite all the guidance and support, I still struggled with illusory fears that sometimes seemed very real to me. *What are the fears and limitations that continue to hold you back in your own spiritual journey? What purpose do they serve? In what way do they offer comfort to the "I" of your small self?*

- Don Sinchi taught me that true happiness is not dependent on outer appearances, and the anchoring memories that connect us to peace and love are mere points of reference—not moments to re-create or fixate on. Our past positive experiences remind us to be in an intimate relationship with the boundless, all-encompassing mystery of love all the time. *In what ways do the happiest memories of your life provide you with a sense of spiritual support? Do you have a tendency to overly fixate on the outer circumstances of those times, or can you see the eternal truths they point you toward?*

- Applying an artistic lens to our experiences helps us see beyond the external layers and plumb the depths of mystery, paradox, and the beauty of being human. Don Sinchi once told me that anyone who has ever fallen in love with life becomes "a poet of evolution," capable of attaining the inconceivable—for it's the poetic inspiration that connects us to the essence of being alive. *In what ways have art, poetry, and other forms of expression helped you connect with your true essence?*

CHAPTER 9

THE HUACHUMA
CEREMONY

A few days later, Don Sinchi came to my hut to announce that my initiation was to continue the following morning—this time, through another sacred plant teacher that was not from the immediate area but from the Andes. "I had a vision that this particular plant spirit is calling to help strengthen your link with Mother Nature. You are now ready to see her more objectively, which will help you further embody the ancestral wisdom."

I was curious about how Don Sinchi was connected to a tradition that was so far from his rainforest home. He explained that the whole continent was once a cradle for ancient and advanced civilizations. What was called the Andes today was once referred to as *Antis*. People who lived in those areas called the Amazon rainforest people the *Atls*. Putting these two names together brought one to the ancient advanced civilization of Atlantis, which I'd read about in mystical texts. Given the powers the ancestors were capable of in so many mystical texts across the globe, such as telepathy and teleportation, I shared with Don Sinchi that it seemed as if they really could have coordinated their efforts to help humanity across the globe.

Don Sinchi smiled affirmatively. "The original ancestors were powerful beings, capable of amazing feats that would defy our imagination today. Huge monuments were left to us as a reminder of that time and the kind of power ancient people possessed. The Nazca lines, Machu Picchu, Chavín de Huántar, and the monoliths of Lake Titicaca are all evidence of human potential that was realized by those long gone. Here in the Amazon as well many discoveries are being made to this day.

"As I shared with you, Romancito, one of the original interdimensional portals, through which the enlightened ancestors came in and out of this world, was called Paititi. When the conquistadors came to this area, they heard about Paititi, but without understanding its true meaning, they mistook it for El Dorado—a place referred to as the 'city of gold.' They never really understood with their primitive minds the timeless value of spiritual gold, to which the real meaning of the name El Dorado alludes.

"A pre-Incan myth mentions Paititi, and the various Amazonian tribal legends confirm it. The Incas visited this area quite often for that reason and exchanged plant medicines, practices, and initiations with the Amazonian people. The Amazonian people were greatly respected in the past for being the guardians of the portal to Paititi. The Yahua nation was connected to the Incas, and there are many Kichwa words in our language to this day."

"Were the Amazonian ancestors guarding a certain knowledge or wisdom that would activate the portal of Paititi?" I asked.

He explained that the original ancestors were beings of great light. Before they left, they invoked the wisdom of the Seven Sisters (Pleiades). In this part of the world, the wisdom of the Seven Sisters was deeply connected to the first sacred plant medicines that helped people remember their cosmic origin.

"My elders shared this legend with me from the end of the enlightened era: A meteorite came down to Earth carrying all the main sacred plants as a helpful reminder for difficult times ahead. It was sent by our ancestors from the Seven Sisters. The last beings of light received this express delivery and taught our people how to use its evolutionary contents as skillful instruments of living wisdom that would stretch throughout the millennia, from one human to another: chieftains to tribes, healers to patients, and sorcerers to apprentices."

Don Sinchi explained that these living wisdom lineages were given to humanity as catalysts for healing, spiritual evolution, and reactivation of our primordial nature. The evolutionary potential of humankind, filled with the purest intentions, was the only key that could open the portal of Paititi.

The Huachuma medicine was part of an ancient tradition that dates back thousands of years before the Incan civilization. Similar to Ayahuasca, Huachuma was utilized in the Andes as a conduit for ancestral transmissions within various Indigenous mystery schools. This sacred medicine was a major influence in the Tiahuanaco, Wari, Moche, Chavín, Mochica, Nazca, and many other civilizations throughout antiquity.

The Huachuma cactus also goes by the more modern name of San Pedro. I learned that the story behind the San Pedro cactus dates back to the 15th century, when the first missionaries arrived in South America. They encountered many native healers and partook in the ceremonies of various sacred plant medicines, including Huachuma. The effects that the Catholic priests experienced with Huachuma were nothing short of miraculous, and many found great healing and illumination. They also witnessed the native people being healed from severe illnesses through what appeared to be divine intervention. Some of the monks abandoned the Catholic faith as a result of the holy rupture they experienced in themselves, and they wholeheartedly embraced the spirituality of the Amazonians.

The priests who returned soon after to Rome reported to the Pope their discovery of a miraculous plant they named in honor of Saint Peter (San Pedro). According to them, this plant medicine, akin to the biblical Saint Peter, held the key to heaven. Of course, one had to know how to use the key and where the door was, but there was a lot of commotion around this sacred plant in the Vatican at the time.

Upon hearing the missionaries' accounts of healing through a direct connection with the Holy Spirit, the Pope became enraged— maybe out of fear that he would no longer be needed. Not wanting any competition, especially not from a plant, the Pope ordered his people to erase San Pedro from the face of the Earth, alongside all the native "witch doctors" who communed with it. Of course, the Andean healers instantly discovered the Pope's devious plan and hid high in the mountains. Simultaneously, the plant grew in such abundance all over the Andes that even the Pope could not eliminate it from the face of the Earth. The name *San Pedro* stuck, and many native healers today still refer to this plant medicine as such, to commemorate the victory of Mother Nature over persecution.

I was struck that the Andean people applied the same strategy as many other ancient traditions who'd hidden the ancient mystery traditions behind the more commonly acceptable religions of the time. Similarly, here in the Amazon, Don Sinchi sometimes referred to the ceremonies of Ayahuasca as the intimate life of Jesus Christ. All the trials and tribulations, as well as the blessings of the divine that are described in the Bible, could be experienced directly through the sacrament of Ayahuasca.

As he blew a stream of smoke high into the air, Don Sinchi continued, "Although San Pedro does not grow in the jungle, I was initiated into this tradition in my youth. Contrary to many of today's curanderos, who work with only one sacred plant teacher, in ancient times the healers utilized many sacred plants. I got to know the Seven Sisters of the star people through the following plants: Toé, Huachuma, Ayahuasca, Huillca, Mama Coca, Mapacho, and the sacred Kajampa mushrooms. Different healers may connect with the enlightened ancestors from the realm of the Seven Sisters through other sacred plants that are relevant to their lineages as well."

I learned that the number seven held special significance for many tribes, especially for the Yahuas. In their cosmovision, there were seven celestial levels of mastery on the journey through the ocean of the Great Spirit to the star people of Paititi. The diverse sacred plant lineages the ancients worked with also corresponded to the seven levels of inner discipline: 1) the seed finding the right conditions for opening, 2) germinating, 3) sprouting through the darkness of the underworld into the light, 4) being a tender seedling, 5) then a daring sapling, 6) gradually turning into a wise tree, and finally, 7) becoming a great healer.

"In your healing journey, you are just beginning to sprout onto the first level, from the underworld of self-destructive illness," Don Sinchi explained. "It's essential to take it step by step and thoroughly transmute the unconscious habits of your life."

He explained that each medicinal plant within his ancestral lineage had to be experienced on its own before it was combined with other plants. Some plants, like Huachuma, were dangerous to ingest at the same time as Ayahuasca. Yet, it was beneficial when each was ingested separately and at least a day apart. Ayahuasca catapults you into the source of your creative potential, and Huachuma teaches you to embody that creative potential in everyday life.

"The realization and embodiment of potential is, however, a more advanced level of our living wisdom that you are not ready for yet," Don Sinchi was quick to add. "We are still clearing the debris of your hopes and fears at this time. Whether you are hoping for something to happen or afraid of what might happen, you are not present with the full potential of who you are in each moment. Still, my intuition tells me that the transmission of the Andean mountains might help you gain a higher perspective."

The First Two Gateways

The next day, Don Sinchi awoke me at 7 A.M. and told me we had the whole day to dedicate to the Huachuma medicine.

The elder then gave me a word of caution: "Now, don't you get carried away by laughter during this ceremony. Although the Huachuma spirit has a fresh sense of humor, serious lessons often accompany it—especially if you lose presence. This plant medicine can also magnify all your other emotions. Similar to Ayahuasca, it teaches us how to ride the waves of emotions, sensations, and mental dramas. Getting hooked by the disturbances can cause a serious headache for both the patient and the healer, because he is the one who potty trains the patient's monkey mind. Therefore, today I will guide you through the wisdom of this sacred plant lineage in the same way I was introduced by my Andean elders. The ceremony consists of various gateways, established by the ancestors through thousands of years of connection with Huachuma medicine and cultivation of unwavering focus."

Don Sinchi then spread an offering cloth woven with colorful geometric patterns, a gift from a Shipibo elder, on the ground in front of him. He carefully took out ceremonial items from his woven satchel bag. He then placed decorated stones and etched crystals from the mountains, as well as different local plants, fruits, and vegetables, onto his ceremonial cloth. He shared that the foods he placed on the cloth were essential to the rainforest people and therefore appropriate for the *despacho* (offering) to the Great Spirit. He also placed a handful of mapacho leaves on the altar and refilled his pipe. Finally, the elder took out a bag of dry cactus powder, made a prayer in Yahua, lit his pipe, and blew mapacho smoke infused with his intentions into the sacrament and all over the altar.

We proceeded with the ingestion of the sacrament; I went first. The taste was extremely bitter. Seeing the sour expression on my face, Don Sinchi said with a smile, "It tastes bitter, like the truth."

After about a half hour of silence, he began shaking his rattle and singing his sacred songs. At that point, I started to feel nauseated, weak, and tired all at once. My mind panicked, commanding me to crawl into a corner and forget about the whole thing . . . yet I kept breathing through it, as Don Sinchi had taught me to do.

After some time, Don Sinchi told me we had reached the first gateway; in order to activate it, we had to get up and start circulating the energy through our bodies. Although I didn't feel like it, I got up. He told me that we would practice a series of Andean exercises called *quntur,* or "condor" in the Kichwa language. The condor flies high but can see the tiniest details down on the earth. The practice, I was told, was meant to focus the awareness on being in the moment, which is where the bird's-eye view is found.

We started performing an intricate series of movements—stretching every joint, ligament, and tendon. In some moments, we would stand still in strange postures and vigorously shake our bodies afterward. Several of our movements involved kissing the ground, and some involved hugging a large Wayra Caspi tree that stood nearby. Toward the end of the exercises, we squatted; with our knees up around our ribs, we created internal heat by tapping our knees on our ribs, toward the areas of the liver and pancreas. Upon finishing these exercises, to my great surprise, I felt rejuvenated and lucid, compared to how I'd previously felt.

Don Sinchi sang a few icaros upon completing the exercises, which intensified the effects of the medicine. I was tangibly experiencing the circulation of life force in my body, making me more agile, limber, and present than ever before.

The Rimyurá then told me we were entering the second gateway, which entailed a walk into the rainforest. As I followed Don Sinchi deeper into the wilderness, Nature appeared more glorious to me. The foliage that surrounded us sparkled with vibrant colors. Through my own breath, I could feel all the life-forms surrounding me, breathing in unison as one conscious organism. I was simultaneously conscious of everyone and everything in the rainforest, just as I could experience the arms and legs connected to my physical body in everyday life.

After about an hour of venturing deeper into the rainforest, we stopped by a tremendous White Lupuna tree that seemed to be about 100 feet in diameter. Don Sinchi had introduced me to this tree before, calling it the king of all trees and a wise teacher of the spiritual path. As we sat, sheltered by the shade of the giant tree, Don Sinchi made a mapacho offering by blowing smoke from his pipe onto the roots of the tree beneath our feet. He then sang a few icaros to connect the medicine spirit within us to the spirit of the tree. I sat in anticipation of what would happen next.

The Third Gateway

After settling by the Lupuna tree, Don Sinchi told me that a third gateway activation was approaching, in which we would engage in a special breath practice that some tribes utilize in their ceremonies as part of an energetic cleanse. I followed his instructions, and we took deep diaphragmatic breaths that gradually intensified as we shook our bodies to the rhythm of our breath.

While exhaling, Don Sinchi made the soft "ha" sounds I recognized from my welcoming rite of passage into the Yahua tribe. He also instructed me to focus on different energy centers in the body, starting from the tailbone all the way to the top of the head, and to relate them to various elements of nature while we synchronized our breathing rhythms. I recognized that these were similar to the chakras in the Vedic system: elemental vortexes that could help us access great energy.

The longer I kept up with the rhythmic breathing, the more I felt my body release trapped energies at each center—especially the water one in my belly that corresponded to the location of my sickness. Emotions of sadness, frustration, and self-judgment emerged from the source of my physical disharmony. As I kept breathing into the bothersome areas of my being, the pent-up emotions were shaken out of my body with cathartic convulsions. The breathwork was expelling all the stagnation from me, like dust beaten out of a rug.

As we reached the throat center, we both started jumping up and down, while breathing deeply and quickly. Reality was filled with bright sparks of light, just as I remembered from my early childhood. I began dissolving into the brilliance of the rainforest. Simultaneously, I experienced the same bright energy erupting from inside me. Inside and outside merged. My body ceased to exist, and my consciousness lost all sense of time and space.

We kept breathing increasingly faster while focusing on the forehead, immersing into the intensifying luminosity of the all-encompassing life force. When we reached the top of the head, we both harmonized and hummed a buzzing sound. In that moment, the sound we made together turned into a tremendous swarm of bees. Light surged through my core, piercing the molecular and possibly genetic structure of my DNA.

We then began to gradually slow our breath, focusing on bringing the energy down, center by center, landing from another dimension until we reached Earth. At the end of the practice, we let out a primal scream, releasing whatever stagnation still remained in our bodies. Right after that, we sat quietly to observe the deeper awakening, which the plant medicine, coupled with the breathwork practice, had catalyzed within us. The results of that breathwork were remarkable; I became one with all of creation and felt like I was blissfully bursting with the vibrational forces of Nature within.

At a certain point during that timeless meditation, Don Sinchi began to speak in a quiet, assertive, melodious tone: "What you are experiencing right now is inherent to all beings' state of truth. The truth of our being is neither bleak nor static. It's an omnipresent blissful state of existence that does not depend on extremes of pleasure or pain. Such joyous bliss is not here for us to get lost and indulge in, or else we'll sink back into delusion. Truth is naturally selfless and is all about sharing presence in compassionate reciprocity with an infinitely vast universe. The truth of your own heart-centered awareness is your unshakable anchor of harmony that illuminates the furthest, deepest, darkest corners of the universe."

Unlike so many of my previous experiences, in which Don Sinchi's tendency to speak in riddle and rhyme only served to confuse me, I could finally understand what the elder was saying—not only with my conceptual mind, but also with my entire being. I closed my eyes to root more deeply into this moment of truth. What followed was timeless silence, filled with the sound of the rainforest coming alive with myriad life-forms.

After what seemed like an eternity of me being everything and nothing at the same time, the sounds of Don Sinchi's singing and his maraca snapped me back into a solid sense of self. I felt my physical body like never before; every cell vibrated with bliss and love. Just like the elder had described before we started the ceremony, my Ayahuasca ceremonies had propelled me to find lost creative energy in the furthest corners of my inner universe, but Huachuma was now grounding all the facets of my being to unify and blossom within my physical body.

Don Sinchi finished singing and motioned me to come closer. I sat in front of the elder. He told me to remain quiet and look into his eyes while softening my body first, then my face, and finally my gaze. I followed his directions and, upon meeting his nighthawk eyes, experienced something inexplicable. It was similar to experiencing a blackout when standing up too fast, but instead of darkness, I experienced the light of a thousand suns. I lost my identity, and yet, without anyone there that I could call "myself," I found the pure rupture of omniscient presence. Nothing dissolved into Everything. No body, no center, no borders. No rainforest, no Roman, no Don Sinchi. No thoughts, no mind, no limits. What remained was beyond words. There was just a timelessly radiant presence of primordial love. When I finally opened my eyes after what seemed to be an eternity, Don Sinchi was nowhere in sight.

There I was, alone, in the presence of the benevolent 1,000-year-old Lupuna tree, encircled by the vast rainforest, experiencing itself through me. I stayed there, basking in the warm embrace of Nature until sunset. As it got darker, the hungry hordes of mosquitoes sent me stumbling back to Don Sinchi's house, somehow intuitively guided through the rainforest trails I vaguely recognized.

Tool: Unlocking Your Energetic Vortexes

Tune in to the way your body feels at different energy centers: lower back, hips, belly, solar plexus, chest, throat, and head. What elements do you associate with each of these areas? Be creative by coming up with any ways you can loosen up and be more at ease with yourself and the world. Standing up, breathing loudly, screaming, and tremoring may seem irrational and ridiculous to the conceptual monkey mind, but consider the possibility that our rigid mental habits, such as being preoccupied with our image, are a lot more ridiculous. With the help of physical practices that shake and move stagnant energy, you can learn to ride the stormy waves of your emotions without being swept away by them.

The Tender Medicine of the Deer

My teacher was waiting for me back at the house with a delicious dinner made by Warmi, which, unlike the Ayahuasca dieta, had a lot of flavor. While we ate, Don Sinchi took the opportunity to share more about the healing journey of transformation: "Nature is constantly communicating to us, but it's a different language than the one we are used to in human society. It's a language of uncontainable life force that gracefully flows through each organism. I see that you are beginning to understand it, even though your mind is still somewhat resistant to the wisdom of your body."

I asked him to explain what he meant.

"Remember I once told you about all life-forms being the channels of Mother Earth and Father Sun? This rabbit hole goes deeper yet," he said. "Evolutionary Science states that our essential nature is to be conscious channels of Universal Love. All the imbalances, sicknesses, and 'dis-eases' stem from us dwelling in the illusion of separation from that eternal flow."

He went on to explain that the breathwork practice we did earlier in the day was one of the ancient tools that helps activate both the energy flow within us and the wisdom of our organisms to channel it harmoniously. The ancients called it the *Huayra-Otorongo* ("wind jaguar" in Kichwa) wave. One of the reasons for that name is that the hands and feet can sometimes feel like they're turning into claws.

"As you may remember from your Yahua welcoming, the tribes of the rainforest trace their origin to cats rather than monkeys, which is where modern people must think they come from, with their monkey minds," said Don Sinchi.

The breathwork we'd done tapped into the power of the jaguar's heart in our very own being. It is still practiced extensively in the Orinoco basin of the Amazon by the Yanomami tribe. Don Sinchi explained that he'd been initiated into it at a young age by a Huitoto elder. The Yahuas have been practicing it in their tribe ever since.

"How does this wave practice combine with the other waves you introduced me to?" I asked.

"All of the wave practices are unified by profound insights into the multifaceted wisdom of Mother Nature. The Huayra-Otorongo practice originated when the Yanomami ancestors witnessed a deer escaping the claws of a jaguar. Once that deer found safety, it began breathing in distinct patterns that alternated every few minutes. The rhythmic breath of the animal was accompanied by shakes and tremors that helped it release all the accumulated anxiety and fear. As all the stress trapped in its body from the traumatic encounter with the jaguar was released, the deer suddenly became infused with incandescent luminosity, which pulsated from its heart. That deer was a divine messenger of Nature's intelligence and has since become the Yanomamis' sacred symbol of the heart's wisdom. Other tribes, including ours, also honor the deer spirit as an animal totem that represents the tender, loving medicine of the heart.

"The embodiment of deer wisdom necessitates an unwavering determination of the deer's heart to unite the opposites: the humility of the monkey mind and the guidance of the spiritual lineage. The enlightened ancestors of the Yanomamis, with their insight into the true nature of reality, followed a lineage that directly engages our cellular memory, which is woven energetically throughout our physical bodies, not just the head."

As Don Sinchi shared, according to the Yanomamis, certain memories in our lives are pushed deep under the surface of our waking existence and into the underworld of hungry, ferocious demons. The memories trapped there are initially inaccessible to the first wave of remembrance practice. However, the primordial breathwork that Don Sinchi had shared with me is capable of awakening pure presence, untainted by the sense of "me" and "mine." The practice, when done wholeheartedly and consistently, infuses the breath of life into the cellular memory of the body over time, helping one access trapped memories and their associated emotions and sensations.

The full story of our lives can be found in our entire bodies, not just our heads—a lesson I was beginning to integrate. The body naturally knows what the original anchor of well-being is, because we all come from the womb of Mother Nature. The body also knows all the tensions and contractions that guard our original state of innocent well-being from being hurt by the harsh realities of the modern world. The physical organism always abides in the present moment and constantly engages the energy of thoughts, emotions, and sensations, even when the mind is distracted.

Don Sinchi continued, "When the awareness is present in the body, without shying away from the energies of each moment, whether pleasurable or painful, the body begins to remember what it means to be a channel. That is what's known as the energy body: a connecting link between the everyday awareness of one's biological self and the dreaming realm of one's spirit. Gradually becoming conscious of the life force flowing through one's organism chips away at the resistance to life on deeper and deeper levels. As you become more open to life, you naturally tap into the realm of the Great Spirit and the loving wisdom of Mother Nature."

The Monkey and the Jaguar

"Can you share some of that wisdom, Don Sinchi?"

"Remember that Nature's wisdom is not conceptual. It is the wisdom of our organism, and it manifests in our inner wellness, receptivity, and wholehearted relatedness—all those essential qualities that are the cornerstones of every culture on Earth. Our people see these qualities as essential for humanity because they are the qualities that all human beings get to know while in the Mother's womb—cradled in the waters of creation, fully supported and provided for, while blissfully abiding in a state of no separation between the consciousness of the Mother and the Child. That is the original happiness of interconnectedness everyone is intuitively trying to get back to. Different people may have different ideas in terms of how to reach happiness, but the happiness itself is beyond definition. Happiness, for our people, is that original cellular memory embedded in the core of all living organisms that we all intuitively know yet can never fully describe."

Unfortunately, as Don Sinchi explained, once we emerge from the Great Mother's womb, we begin to experience all the disturbing emotions that involve separation from our original anchor state. Consequently, innocence gets associated with woundedness—especially because there isn't a place in modern society for innocence and vulnerability.

Don Sinchi paused and began mimicking the modern mentality: "If I am innocent and vulnerable, someone can hurt me and take advantage of me! It's safer for me to develop a thick skin and pretend to be just like everyone else!"

He looked piercingly at me and continued, "In our Indigenous culture, however, essential human qualities that are based on profound values, like innocence, are indispensable when it comes to remembering ourselves as open channels of Universal Love. Even our wounding around our innocence, when it's embraced through Mother Nature's wisdom, becomes a healing portal that can awaken the unconditional presence of the heart."

He stopped talking, pointing out a tribe of monkeys swinging through the treetops above us while screeching and hollering.

"Would you refer to woundedness as conditioning, Don Sinchi?" I asked, unimpressed by the monkeys above us.

"Woundedness is not conditioning in and of itself, but how we relate to it can be. Imagine for a moment that the human organism is a very advanced, finely tuned spaceship, designed for interdimensional travel." He paused and grinned mischievously. "Are you surprised that I talk about spaceships?"

I responded that I was getting used to him being full of surprises. He giggled and went on, "Within this magnificent spaceship, however, sits our monkey mind. Hollering, grunting, and screaming, this belligerent monkey breaks all the fine-tuned cosmic instruments by pressing all the wrong buttons."

He burst out laughing at his own image for a few minutes, echoing the loud sounds of the monkeys until they moved out of our hearing range. "The process of healing and evolution is directly related to that monkey in the spaceship. And by no means do we want to annihilate the monkey. The untrained monkey mind is a capricious master, who only cares about superficial and instant gratification as a way to avoid the emotional woundings of life."

As Don Sinchi spoke, I realized that becoming a humble steward of Mother Nature, wholeheartedly dedicated to the shared heart of all beings, was one of the best ways we could fully heal wounded innocence. Such transformation took place by training the mind to listen to the subtle life force behind our noisy everyday thoughts. The broken record of the mind's ranting had no meaning whatsoever most of the time, anyway.

Don Sinchi explained that this was a huge realization for the ancestors: that instead of filling our heads with the garbage of social conditioning, we could infuse our whole being with prayers consciously expressed through every breath. Icaros were such a practice. The healing songs were the culmination of many generations invoking their highest purpose. The light of ancestral intentions was rewoven into the sacred breath of life via the reverberations of the Great Spirit.

"Remembering the nature within us through the melodies of our ancestors realigns the distorted life force within," he said.

"What about the ego, then, which makes us feel so separate from nature?" I asked.

"The ego is the monkey mind I am referring to. Contrary to many modern belief systems, it's essential to life. Without the ego, we wouldn't be able to talk, walk, eat, or perform some of life's most essential basic functions. However, the ego must know its place. The mind needs much training to humbly express the universal qualities of our organism, instead of distorting Nature to fit its own self-absorbed conditioning. Evolution begins with the realization that the ego plays an essential, but not the most important, role. This whole time you have been here has been a preparation for you to start potty training your monkey mind."

Although I must've sounded ridiculous with all my questions, it was more important for me to understand than to fear looking like a fool. I still didn't fully get the connection between the ego and our fundamental innocence, so I asked Don Sinchi to elaborate.

"When the child lacks support and guidance, the innocence is wounded. As a result, the inspiration to evolve gets lost in the illusion of appearances and becomes trapped by fear. In the absence of genuine unconditional love, the mind clings to appearances like an infant who clutches their security blanket. Wounded innocence, left unresolved, gets covered by belief systems that offer false protection from illusory monsters under the bed. Animalistic survival, self-gratification, and personal ambition gradually take precedence over essential human values. These tendencies eventually develop into the unruly monkey mind, which tyrannically rules over the heart by resisting our life experience."

Don Sinchi winced miserably, placing both hands over his heart. "If I open my heart, it will get hurt again, just like last time, so I'd rather never open it again. It's for my own good to be comfortably numb and not feel any pain. I believe that the pain is greater than love. I sacrifice love and shut the heart, so I won't be punished by my master, The Pain."

Witnessing the elder's charade, I got the clear sense that he was accurately mirroring my inner state of affairs, whereby my mind tends to rule my life, making me fear my own vulnerability. The elder suddenly stopped mimicking and looked at me with a cunning smile.

"Those are but some of the many tricks that our own minds play on us. As our innocence is healed, however, Nature's creative power becomes liberated, allowing us to evolve from childish to childlike. When we grow out of our destructive infantile behavior, there's no longer a need to unconsciously feed on artificial substitutes for our aliveness. The uncontainable forces of nature that seemed so scary before suddenly reveal their healing potential—by pointing out the boundless, loving essence beneath all appearances. The child begins to play intelligently, with a higher purpose in sight."

The Rimyurá's gesticulations transformed into graceful expressions; he was almost dancing as he expanded further on the subject: "The evolutionary healing path gradually transforms the monkey mind from a capricious master into a humble devotee of the heart. No longer distrusting the heart's unconditional wisdom, the mind discovers its true purpose, which is to help awaken fearless love under all circumstances. As you familiarize yourself with the path I am guiding you along, more specific details about this training will be revealed."

He suddenly got up and gave me a strong hug that I didn't expect from someone his age. He then told me that after a Huachuma ceremony, a long, good rest is essential—and that breakfast would be ready for me when I awoke in the morning.

I went back to my hut and stayed wide awake deep into the night. It was impossible to sleep with the Great Spirit speaking loudly through the lively, enchanted rainforest . . . because I was finally beginning to understand the Spirit's language with my entire being.

Tool: Hugging the Tree of Life

Here's a Quntur practice that is similar to a Taoist Qigong posture and that can help you still your monkey mind and awaken the jaguar's heart within.

Stand up straight, with knees slightly bent and feet pointed straight, parallel to each other and a bit wider than shoulder width apart. Distribute your weight evenly through the soles of your feet while visualizing roots growing from the soles of your feet into the earth, making you feel more grounded. Pull the tailbone inward to avoid stress on the lower back.

Use your arms to make a big circle, with a small distance between your hands in front of your chest. Make the circle in your upper back as well, like a barrel expanding in all directions from the center of your chest. Keep your shoulders relaxed, chest open, and body at ease. Start with 10 minutes and gradually increase the duration.

It may be challenging to hold this position at first, but it will become easier over time when you do the practice without engaging the monkey mind. You will also feel a greater sense of vitality. Remind yourself that this is not a strength exercise but a trust exercise; that is, you're learning to trust the space of the heart to support you through life's challenges.

Pay attention to your breath and the optimal position of your body in the posture. The static meditative positions are known in Amazonian, Andean, and Eastern cultures to be highly beneficial for humbling the monkey mind and connecting to the life force within. If you don't mind the tensions, minor aches, and discomforts throughout the practice, your energy channels will open and your tensions will transform.

REFLECTIONS

- Don Sinchi shared the experience of the Catholic priests of the 15th century witnessing the ways in which the Indigenous people were healed from illness through "divine intervention" when they ingested the sacred plant medicine of Huachuma. Many of them ended up embracing Evolutionary Science and abandoning their dogmatic faith. I experienced something similar as the grip of my conceptual mind gave way to a deeper understanding that came through my heart, which helped me recognize the aliveness of the world around me in ways I'd never previously known. *Have you experienced moments of "holy rupture" in your life—when an existing belief system was shattered by Nature revealing herself to you?*

- Don Sinchi helped me see and understand that the energy body isn't something that lives "outside" of us—it's the intermediary between our biology and our spirit. It's the experience of recognizing that our body has the ability to channel all experiences as pure life force. *When have you most keenly felt the full spectrum of your own life force? How did you feel about this, and how did it help you chip away at resistance or fear-based thinking?*

- Many of us are attempting to get back to an "original happiness" that is deeply intertwined with a wholeness that lives inside our cellular memory and is connected to the experience of being held in the warm, loving womb of Mother Nature. *What are the substitutes you've attempted to use to get back to that original happiness? And what are the times in your life when you've felt most connected to that original happiness—not based on pleasure versus pain but outside of and beyond external circumstances or desires?*

- Don Sinchi perfectly encapsulated the modern mentality that keeps us from feeling and honoring our own vulnerability: we fear opening the heart because we associate this with memories of being hurt. We are conditioned by our experiences and by the world around us to keep our heart closed so that we'll avoid feeling pain, believing this pain is greater than love. *Think of your own relationship with vulnerability. In what ways has your innocence been wounded? What decisions did you make with respect to opening and closing your heart? What were the costs and benefits associated with closing your heart? In what ways are you learning to keep it open?*

CHAPTER 10

THE QUEST FOR A BLESSING FROM THE PINK DOLPHINS

The day after the Huachuma ceremony, Don Sinchi called me into the maloka. Once I settled on the floor next to the elder, he informed me that the ceremony I'd just been through had been an initial introduction to the Huachuma plant teacher. Don Sinchi said I'd demonstrated a deep affinity for the plant medicine, so it would be appropriate for me to go through a deeper rite of passage with it. In the Huachuma tradition, there was a special initiation involving a pilgrimage to sacred places and the magical beings that abided in them.

"Will you accept the invitation of the Spirit to embark on such a journey?" The elder looked inquisitively at me.

I told him that I would, of course, be honored. He then shared that as part of the initiation I was to embark on, alongside his nephew Chispa, into the rainforest, I was supposed to seek out the blessing of the *bufeos colorados*—or pink dolphins. These dolphins operated on a similar frequency as the spirit of Huachuma and were revered throughout the Amazon as wise beings, imbued with mystical powers. For that purpose, the Rimyurá provided me with a large, fresh Huachuma cactus and specific instructions on how to prepare it; I was to slice the cactus into many pieces, then wrap all of them in newspaper and wait for a week for them to turn into a viscous substance. The plant preparation had to start before journeying to our final destination.

Don Sinchi told me we were going to visit Porfirio, an old friend of his far up the river Yarapa, one of the rivers that empties into the Amazon. Once I got there, I would dry whatever was left of the cactus in the sun before ingesting it. The ceremony was to be conducted in the presence of the pink dolphins. Only if I was successful—meaning that I'd drink the medicine upon arrival at my destination and easily commune with the pink dolphins—would I become initiated into that tradition and be allowed to learn it.

I immediately began the initial preparation of the cactus and carefully wrapped it in newspaper. A few days later, Chispa and I set out on our journey. According to my calculations as I studied the map, Porfirio—who lived a few days away, near a village called Libertad—was about 250 miles from us. Chispa shared with me that he has been trying to become Don Sinchi's apprentice without much luck for a while, and this quest was his opportunity to deepen his studies with the elder.

The barge we got onto had a big motor and an open, roofless deck, covered with hundreds of hammocks and a multitude of passengers occupying them. People were sleeping, listening to radios, and talking over the constant, loud rumbling of the motors that slowly propelled us, first down the Tahuayo River and then up the Yarapa River. I tried not to be discouraged by the chaos of the people and the noisy motor, instead focusing on the beautiful scenery; I was in awe of the ancient trees, which became even more colossal the farther upriver we went. The foliage that leaned over the river provided a pleasant shade from the intense heat.

Despite my best efforts, I was still bothered by the loud engines, so I decided to try and channel my disturbances into the wave of remembrance practice that Don Sinchi had taught me. Since Don Sinchi had encouraged me to begin working with difficult childhood memories, I figured I could use the chaotic boat ride as a point of reference to trace my earliest experiences of feeling "disturbed."

I started to implement the breathing technique the elder had taught me. With each breath, I gradually immersed myself in the experiences of my faintly outlined early trauma, first vaguely, and gradually, more vividly.

The Beginning of Patterns of Suffering

I remembered myself at the age of three, which was a crucial threshold in my development. Both my parents, despite their differences, loved me. Their attitude and approach to raising me, however, differed substantially. I was a difficult child, mirroring the growing discord between my parents. My mother, who was already struggling with her marital issues, would become frustrated with me at times and direct my father to do something about it. That something, according to my mother's own tough upbringing, involved a strong masculine hand with a leather belt in it.

My father, who'd experienced the pointlessness of physical punishment himself as a child, had a different view as to how my life should unfold. He would enter my room with a belt in his hand, shut the door loudly, and quietly instruct me to cry as hard as I could, while he loudly hit the wall with a belt. We would conduct this performance, trying not to giggle in the process, for the benefit of my mother, who was listening intently from the other room.

After this memory unfolded, I was transported to a party my parents organized at our house with their friends during that period of my childhood. Just as before, with the anchor of well-being, I was there once again, reexperiencing those distant events as if they were unfolding in the present: I could see many guests gathered at our home; some of them sat in our backyard at a big table, and others hung out in the living room of our small house. My mother, as an art teacher, had many bohemian friends—musicians, artists, writers. Many creative and artistic types often visited us because we lived on the outskirts of a big city, in the charming countryside. There was music and wine, people dancing and chatting, and then . . . there was me—the only child at the event.

An hour or so into the party I got bored and went to my room. Coming through the open door unnoticed, I overheard my father talking to my mother about leaving. I felt a tangible pain in my gut. It was the first time I knew something was seriously wrong between my parents. I went back out to the yard, where I had a little hiding place in the bushes. I had stashed matches there and would occasionally light a hollow straw, pretending to smoke cigarettes, like my parents did. Now looking back, that night felt like my first smoking prayer. I squeezed out of the hiding place, feeling much calmer, and went to my room, eventually falling asleep to the loud music of the party.

In the morning, I woke up and smelled smoke coming through my window from the outside. Looking out the window, I saw our half-burned backyard. It turned out that my straw ritual had almost burned down our house and scarred half our backyard! While I was peacefully asleep, my parents and their drunk guests were up all night, trying to extinguish the fire I had started. That was my first (unintentional) alchemical fire purification . . .

A few days later, I collapsed from a terrible stomach pain. The doctors suspected meningitis, and my parents took me to the hospital for a spinal tap, despite the fact that it was known to be a dangerous procedure. The spinal tap ruled out meningitis, leaving my stomach pain unexplained. From then on, I experienced random stomachaches, which for a long time were labeled by the doctors and my parents as "growing pains."

Years later, my gastroenterologist mentioned that because Crohn's disease is a genetic condition, the first episodes often begin in early childhood and may remain undiagnosed for a long time.

Soon after that, the growing certainty in my gut proved to be correct. My parents separated, and my father moved out of our family home. For some time, I lived there alone with my mother. I only had a mosaic of my name that my father inlaid into the front porch cement from broken ceramic tiles when I was born to remind me of our once-happy family. Undeterred by my previous experience with fire, my favorite way to pass the time continued to be watching things burn. I loved igniting old newspapers, which I'd retrieve from an old wooden closet that stood outside the front door of our house. I could sit there mesmerized by the fire for hours on end.

Every so often, my father came to visit; during those times, he and my mother would ask me to play outside with my friends. On one such occasion, as I was immersed in fire gazing, my parents requested that I visit my friends. I blew on the fire to extinguish it and went to hang out with my buddies, who lived nearby. I came back a couple hours later, only to discover the whole front of our house on fire, once again. My parents had been so involved in their argument that they didn't even notice the house they were in was ablaze!

I felt guilty for starting yet another fire, and instead of calling my parents for help, I tried to blow it out myself. In a futile attempt to put out the fire, I spit on the raging flames, which kept rising higher and higher into the sky. Finally, my parents came to their senses when they heard the crackling of the fire, smelled the burning, and saw the smoke coming in. They ran outside to see what was happening and found me bravely spitting into a raging inferno. After many buckets of water, the fire was finally put out. Now, seeing this situation from a fresh perspective, that fire was a clear symbol of the emotional turmoil everyone in my family was going through at the time. Our household was falling apart, as our family values were being razed to the ground.

During my father's next visit, he told me that he wanted to take me on a vacation to the sea—just me and him. I was enamored by that idea. My father then went to my mother to get her permission. They began to argue and, as they did before, asked me to play outside with my friends. This time, however, I stubbornly remained to see what would happen. They got into a big argument, which heated up to the point that it got physical. I could no longer bear seeing my loved ones fight; I ran off, screaming and crying. On the way, I saw our neighbors sitting on a bench outside their house. Sobbing, I asked them to help my parents. I then dashed into the nearest bushes, where I felt safe enough for my emotions to settle.

Following that event, my parents went through a lengthy divorce process, fighting over custody of me in court. My mother won and I ended up living with her, while my father was only allowed Sunday visitations.

Soon after, another man moved into our house. Because he was a complete stranger to me, I was encouraged daily by my mother to refer to him as my father. At the same time, my mom had her share of resentment toward my biological father; every time I did something wrong, she reprimanded me by saying that I was just as bad as my father. Being a small, naive child, I became an instrument of revenge between my parents. My father came to visit me every Sunday without fail, just to hear how much I hated him and never wanted to see him again.

It wasn't until now, swinging in a hammock to the sound of rumbling barge motors, that I finally saw how that situation had caused widespread suffering in our family. Consequently, my mother was diagnosed with a nervous system disorder, I ended up with Crohn's disease, and my father went through multiple heart attacks over the years following his separation from my mom.

That session of the wave of remembrance cleared up many stagnant emotions in my being, allowing me to enter the most profound, heart-centered state of peace, clarity, and compassion. I could finally see that no one had ever taught my mom and dad how to be parents. Being human, first and foremost, they were on their own evolutionary journeys, and they had naturally made many mistakes in the process.

I began to understand that the ignorance within people is what causes suffering—not the people themselves. I could finally identify a unique expression of that same ignorance in my own life as the real cause of my suffering; I expected my parents to be perfect and resented them for not meeting my high expectations. Seeing in such a visceral way how hurt people hurt people, I no longer wished to be an unconscious link in the human chain reaction by projecting my unresolved issues onto others.

This became the greatest motivation on my path going forward: to heal myself so that I would no longer inadvertently hurt others. Only by healing myself could I encourage people in my life to heal themselves as well.

Tool: Blessings in Disguise

Once you can maintain the positive anchor of well-being steadily within the wave of remembrance practice, make it a practice to engage your most challenging memories. Once the emotional reactions are disentangled from the challenging memory, objectivity and a bird's-eye view may provide clear insight into a situation that may have appeared negative in the moment but was actually a blessing in disguise when you look back now. After the practice, contemplate how what seems to be a problem in your life right now may also be a blessing in disguise on your evolutionary path. Even though you may not see exactly how the current adversity is a blessing, apply the anchor of well-being to your experience of that adversity, which may help bring about a new realization. You may also begin to identify patterns around similar adversities and your reactions to them—write them down.

The Ordeal with the Mosquitoes

Three days into the river journey, I decided to glance for the first time into the mysterious newspaper with the medicine wrapped in it. To my great dismay, I discovered that the Huachuma hadn't just melted into a simple viscous substance, as I thought it would, but had become rotten and was starting to smell awful. It didn't seem to be an accident, either. It was a logical outcome to the strange recipe given to me by Don Sinchi. I doubted at that point that I'd be able to ingest the rotten slime forming inside the newspaper, even after drying it in the sun.

When I showed Chispa my rotten treasure, he outrightly declined to have anything to do with the vile substance. Blaming everything on my incorrect preparation, he decided to turn our quest into his vacation time.

I attempted to distract myself by enjoying the scenery of the riverbanks. Occasionally, the barge stopped to drop off and pick up passengers in rustic villages along the way. During those brief stops, local women and children would climb aboard, offering all kinds of traditional (exotic to me) foods. These gourmet foods were neatly packaged in plantain leaves, reminding me of elven bread from *The Lord of the Rings*. There was a dish called *juane*, made of rice, one olive, and a hard-boiled egg, molded into a round shape the size of a knuckle and wrapped in banana leaves. Chispa said it represented the head of Saint John (San Juan—hence the name of the dish), and that the optional piece of chicken cost extra because it represented the brain of Christianity. He said that in Catholicism, thinking for oneself came with a hefty price. Chispa ended up buying a few juanes, saying they were safer to eat than fish in the little port villages. His advice made sense to me, and I also got a few, without the chicken.

Then, Chispa found his favorite dish: greasy suri grubs, grilled on a stick. Eating these grubs, like one would a shish kebab, he told me these worms were known to help with constipation and asthma. Seeing the worms reminded me of the goo in my newspaper. I thought that if I could muster enough courage to try one, maybe there was a chance I could also eat Don Sinchi's rotten goo. Yet, right after the first small bite, I was overcome by such a strong wave of repulsion that I couldn't force myself to take another bite.

Finally, toward the early sunset of the third day, we arrived at our destination in the middle of nowhere on one of the bends in the river. I saw a solitary hut, not far from the riverbank, under the shade of immense trees. Beside the hut, there was no sign of civilization; we found ourselves totally immersed in a prehistoric-looking old-growth rainforest.

We were welcomed by the owner, an older man in rugged clothes with a big toothless smile; he introduced himself as Porfirio. His toothless smile became even wider when he heard that we came bearing Don Sinchi's regards. Unfortunately for us, however, he shared that his relatives had just come to visit him from a distant settlement the previous day and there was no more space for anyone else to stay the night in his small house. It was at that point that we realized a tremendous oversight on our part: both Chispa and I had left our tents and mosquito nets back with the Yahuas. We had the hammocks we swung from in the barge, as each passenger was required to bring their own. Porfirio said that, even without mosquito nets, we'd be comfortable sleeping in our hammocks in the woods. He then pointed out the trees nearby, which were thin enough for us to barely wrap our hammocks around. We were still optimistic at that point and asked our host if there were many mosquitoes in that area at night. He answered that there were very few and smiled disarmingly at us, telling us not to worry.

We securely tied our woven nests, anticipating the first peaceful night of sleep in the wilderness after days of rumbling motor noises in the barge. However, the rainforest seemed to have other plans for us . . .

Never in my life, neither before nor after that night, had I witnessed that many mosquitoes. Hordes of voracious buzzing commandos made the air as thick as butter. There was literally no empty space. We couldn't even open our mouths without droves of mosquitoes flying into them. Both Chispa and I frantically put on whatever clothes we had brought with us.

I had three T-shirts, a long-sleeve shirt, two pairs of pants, a sweater, and a few pairs of socks, yet the mosquitoes relentlessly bit through all these layers. I was even bitten right through the hammock, which I'd desperately wrapped around myself like a burrito. The monstrous creatures weren't even bothered by the toxic mosquito repellent I found in my backpack—which I hadn't had to use prior to this, through all the months of my rainforest stay. After a minute, both Chispa and I desperately looked at each other; aside from the horrible chemical smell of the repellent, it seemed to have no effects and only made the mosquitoes even more ravenous and aggressive.

Chispa, muscular and twice my size, decided to fight for his life. The whole night, he kept twisting, turning, kicking, and swatting the swarms of mosquitoes with all his might. I, on the other hand, realized early on that there was no sense in fighting them. I remembered how, in my recent Huachuma initiation, Don Sinchi and I had sat down after the Huayra-Otorongo breathwork. The elder then began to move his hands closer and farther away from each other, while breathing slowly and deeply at the same time. Imitating him in that ceremony, I was able to enter a profound meditative state. Don Sinchi, noticing how I was intently following his cues, had guided me with a soft, clear voice: "Stop identifying with your reactive monkey mind. Instead, realize that the Breath of Life is who you truly are. By sharing your breath with the entire ecosystem, your own organism becomes an amplifier of the Great Spirit. It's our interconnectedness that makes us rise above even the greatest adversities of life."

That experience of sitting with the Yahua elder under the millennial Lupuna tree turned out to be one of the most profound anchoring memories of my life; instead of identifying with my body, I had become the very air permeating my being, while experiencing the physical body as the miniature version of the greater organism of Nature all around. I had realized myself to be the Breath of Life. The Great Mother of Love and the Great Father of Consciousness had temporarily entrusted me with my physical body so that I could be reborn as loving consciousness. An infinitely spacious presence was born in my core, radiating outward.

The memory from my Huachuma initiation was in such contrast to the experience of being bombarded by mosquitoes that it immediately snapped me out of survival mode. I decided to recreate Don Sinchi's instructions by implementing the wave of remembrance practice. Slowly waving my hands closer and farther apart, I began to take deep breaths with equal intervals between inhales and exhales. Soon enough, I entered a deep meditative state. With my mind quieted down, I could steadily maintain the focus on *having* my body, rather than *being* it. All my effort went into identifying with the breath that was infusing me in every moment. I found myself practicing diligently, because my life seemed to depend on being detached from the continuous onslaught.

At one point, halfway through the night, I heard Chispa desperately blurting while spitting out mosquitoes that entered his mouth, "It's impossible—you kill one and a thousand more come to the funeral."

I encouraged Chispa to stop fighting, but my advice fell on deaf ears. I returned my focus to the breath practice, symbolically waving my hands until I eventually entered a trance state between dream and reality that lasted the rest of the night. To get through especially difficult moments, I imagined how the mosquitoes were purifying all my childhood traumas.

When salvation finally came with the sunrise, both Chispa and I looked like swollen balloons, with every millimeter of our bodies bitten many times over. Eyelids, ears, noses, lips, hands, legs—our entire bodies were red and swollen, leaving us deformed beyond recognition. Chispa tried to get up from his hammock first and instantly collapsed, losing consciousness from the loss of blood. Apparently, fighting the mosquitoes so intensely throughout the entire night was a bad idea; his flexed muscles kept pumping more blood for mosquitoes to suck out of him. Chispa regained consciousness shortly after but was incapacitated due to severe blood loss and had to recover in a reclined position from that point on. He later admitted that his was a hard lesson: honoring the Great Spirit instead of reverting to brute force.

I, on the other hand, felt physically fine, despite being swollen all over and itching like crazy. Not having much else to lose at that point, I was more determined than ever to go through with the crazy quest that Don Sinchi had sent us on. I placed the fermented goo of the Huachuma medicine outside in the light of day and sat for a while, eyeing the festering cactus, which refused to dry in the sun. After some time, the desperation in me reached a new, previously unknown threshold, and I asked for the permission of our host to use his kitchen. Porfirio pointed to a small shack behind the house, and I marched in resolutely. Once inside, I placed a frying pan over the fire and carefully scraped the entire slimy content of my newspaper into it. Even after grilling the rotten cactus for half an hour, it still looked like a big, slimy booger; however, at that point I no longer cared about aesthetics. I separated the menacing slimeball into two halves that seemed manageable enough to swallow. Proceeding to shove them into my throat one by one, I resisted my gag reflex, with my eyes tightly shut.

The Pink Dolphin Empowerment

Right after ingesting the vile goo, I ran into the yard and begged our host to show us the pink dolphins. Although I must have appeared insane, Porfirio graciously agreed, feeling somewhat guilty for what had happened the previous night. We got into his small canoe and started paddling up the river. After about an hour, it started to rain. My guide then commented that we might as well go back, because the dolphins never come out in the rain.

I nodded in defeat, beginning to think this mission had been a total failure from the start. I remembered the Yahua initiation into adulthood that Don Sinchi had once shared with me: the initiate is given an impossible task, destined for failure, just to be unconditionally embraced by the tribe. That made me feel better about the ordeal, yet I was still disappointed.

As we turned the boat around and started to head back, the spirit of Huachuma suddenly awakened in my being, tingling and vibrating on a cellular level. I closed my eyes and drifted into other dimensions, when photographic visions began flooding my inner being: I saw the canoe we were in, but from the bottom of the river. Looking up, I glimpsed a long oval outline of the boat, surrounded by a halo of light. I was rapidly approaching the boat from the river's depths.

The next moment, astounded, I opened my eyes, just in time to see a family of seven pink dolphins jump out of the water and begin dancing around our canoe. The realization that Huachuma had allowed me to see through the dolphins' eyes was baffling. The bufeos colorados were much more massive than their gray ocean cousins, with big, crooked noses. The openings at the tops of their heads, through which they happily exuded fountains of water accompanied by loud woofing noises, made them resemble miniature whales.

I felt the ecstatic presence of the dolphins so strongly that, without giving it a second thought, I stripped off all my clothes and dived into the river, joining their ranks. We were hugging and communing in an interdimensional language, mysteriously unlocked in me by the plant medicine, thus crossing the language barrier between species. The dolphins were telepathically sharing their perception of the universe, introducing a frequency of consciousness so elevated that I sensed only heavenly beings could embody it.

The dolphins shared with me that their purpose on Earth was to hold the vibration of planetary awareness and prevent it from descending into oblivion, despite the ignorance of humankind. Surprisingly, they were not dismayed by us humans. Instead, they had nothing but compassion for us, as we were the lost children of the universe. At that moment, they transformed into a beautiful human family of mama, papa, and child dolphins, swimming around me in a circle, holding hands and rejoicing. I'd previously heard the Amazonian myths in which dolphins had the ability to shape-shift into different forms, but I'd never imagined the myths could be real. The only distinction from being human seemed to be the blowholes atop their heads.

They began to teach me how to work more consciously with the lucid awareness they were transmitting. Rather than indulging in the experience of lightness and ease, I was guided to focus on practical resolution of all my predicaments through more objective and empowering perspectives. The dolphins were reminding me that evolution happens through play, just as I had experienced during my infant years.

I recalled states of being from when I was just learning to walk in life, when toppling over and getting up were equally exciting. Failing would not deter me from continuing to be more creative and intentional about standing up. How could I have forgotten my awe-inspiring disposition to face all challenges in life, which I'd embodied so much as a child?!

My rendezvous with the humanoid dolphins seemed to last an interminable time. As the sun began to set, the enchanted creatures transformed back into their biological forms. In sync, they let out a high-pitched roar, danced around me, and swam away, diving deep into the river and leaping abruptly. Beside myself with joy, I climbed back into the canoe, where my guide was patiently waiting. It was evening, a cue for us to head back. As multicolored clouds were reflected in the flowing waters of the Yarapa River, Porfirio and I began our slow paddle back to his house.

Porfirio later shared with me that he had never seen the wild pink dolphins commune so closely and for such a long time with a human being. Because of legal and illegal mining, the pink dolphins were slowly becoming extinct and were now on the endangered species list. I wondered how many more magical creatures used to exist in the Amazon and the rest of the world before the pandemic of forgetfulness took over.

In the late evening, our friendly host graciously provided both Chispa and me with beds and mosquito nets inside his house. His relatives had boarded a barge to go back to their village earlier that day, probably due to pity for us. However, I was so exhilarated from my communion with the pink dolphins that I couldn't sleep.

The moon was full as I lay in bed, overwhelmed with awe and wonder. I was nearly over the previous night's deathly bout with mosquitoes. It seemed so trivial and petty in comparison to the divine bliss I had just experienced with the pink dolphins. I was ready to undergo dozens of nights with mosquitoes biting me all over just to experience the same Huachuma ceremony all over again.

The next day, Chispa started to regain his vitality, and he was able to walk more easily. I was still concerned for his well-being, so we decided to wait one more day before heading back home. I spent that day swinging gently in my hammock. It was a tremendous blessing to be so deep in the heart of the rainforest, where my heart continued to open in so many wondrous, new ways.

Five days later, I was back at Don Sinchi's abode, relaying all my experiences to him.

The elder had a long, hearty belly laugh as he heard me out. He then confided: "I gave you that specific way of preparing Huachuma to test you and see what you are made of. Of course, there are other, easier ways to prepare and ingest it. However, in this life, we often don't appreciate the blessings if not for the purifications that come beforehand.

"This initiation was a perfect example of it; if it wasn't for the mosquitoes, the bond with the pink dolphins wouldn't have been as strong and their transmission would not have gone as deep. When a human child's innocence is supported, their evolution is accelerated through role-playing, imitation, and interaction. Similarly, the dolphins apply their own innocence to invoke the Great Mother's love, which is expressed through all living beings. It's their intelligent playfulness that allows dolphins to see how disconnected humanity has become. Hence, the compassion that the dolphins showed you for the human predicament on the planet today; the bufeos colorados see humans as lost children trying to find their way back home to unconditional love."

Don Sinchi reminded me of another deep insight I had during that journey: no matter how difficult the purification might seem or actually is, it's insignificant in comparison to the brilliance of our true nature and our inherent capacity for love!

It took Chispa and me about two months to heal fully from the mosquito bites. From that point on, my body became almost immune to the mosquitoes. It seemed that it was just another toll I had to pay on the ancestral highway of alchemical transformation. The elevated consciousness of the dolphins and their otherworldly perception has continued to be a guiding force in my life ever since.

Tool: Attuning to the Pink Dolphins

While the pink dolphins may not be in your vicinity, you can still invoke the frequency of their consciousness by tuning in to your childhood memories of play. Engage the wave of remembrance practice by bringing to mind ways you tackled challenges such as learning to walk. Now apply the same curious, exuberant disposition to your current predicaments. This allows you to simultaneously engage with the wave of remembrance practice of anchoring positive memories while making them immediately applicable to your current adversities.

REFLECTIONS

- The wave of remembrance practice helps us anchor into well-being so we can feel safe and open enough to recognize that the most difficult experiences are also the most important because they are the ones capable of awakening us to our true nature. *Is there a specific anchoring memory that helps you maintain a stable, calm presence whenever you think about it? If so, what is it? How does it make you feel? Can you commit to holding it in your body in the coming days, especially in figuratively stormy weather?*

- All of us go through unpleasant initiations from time to time that test our resilience and take us into our depths. But after the storm comes the rainbow. *Bring to mind any meaningful initiation that came after a period of strife. Did you have any emotional breakthroughs that helped you reframe your challenges and even feel grateful for them?*

- We often forget that other life-forms also have consciousness—and many have consciousness that far surpasses that of the human being in his or her typical habitat! *Have you had any experiences with plants or animals that helped you connect with a more elevated consciousness or understanding?*

CHAPTER 11

THE MASTERY
OF LOVE

Remembering to Dream

Soon after my rite of passage with the pink dolphins, while I was still recovering from the anemia caused by blood loss due to the mosquitoes, Don Sinchi came to visit me. He checked my vitals and invited me to accompany him on a plant-gathering trip through the rainforest. When we approached a small creek, Don Sinchi asked me to sit next to him beside a big Toé plant with beautiful angel trumpet flowers, which had the most divine smell emanating from them.

"Do you know anything about this plant medicine?" he asked.

"Only that it's very sacred, and that many healers fear and respect it," I replied.

"And they are right to do so!"

Don Sinchi told me in no uncertain terms that this plant was not to be messed with. Toé was an ancient medicine and very difficult to navigate consciously. In the Evolutionary Science tradition, one was required to first complete a three-year apprenticeship with Ayahuasca before being initiated into Toé. The only exception was when the medicine was given to someone for specific ailments. It was especially effective with neurological movement disorders, such as a damaged spinal column, epilepsy, and Parkinson's disease, among others.

I'd previously read that the active ingredient was a neurotoxin, but was curious to hear from the elder as to why the medicine was so difficult to navigate.

"Toé directly engages the dreaming force of the Universal Consciousness," Don Sinchi explained. "Although it's still too early for you to work with this medicine directly, you can begin invoking its spirit to support you in the dreaming wave practice I am about to share with you."

I recalled that he'd mentioned the dreaming wave practice back when he'd introduced me to the remembrance practice. I tried to contain the excitement rising from my long period of impatiently waiting for Don Sinchi to share it with me.

He smiled. "How is the wave of remembrance practice going for you, by the way?"

I admitted that although I'd had profound breakthroughs with it, it continued to bring up difficult energies at times, requiring a great amount of effort on my part. I felt exhausted from using up all my resources in the process. However, I wasn't complaining about it; I definitely saw much more clearly all the people in my life with whom I had unresolved tensions, and the circumstances surrounding them. Seeing how damaging the unresolved past continued to be in my life was revealing how much of a messy knot I was on the inside, with no idea how to even begin untangling myself. However, layer by layer, I was slowly releasing the lingering tensions and buried emotions accompanying painful memories, while realizing the higher purpose of all those experiences.

I had traced the earliest origin of my illness back to the time when my parents went through a messy divorce. Even though I was just a child at the time and could not understand what was happening, the atmosphere in our house was so tense it could be cut with a knife. Experiencing that stress on an energetic level and without any understanding turned me into a difficult child. I had emotional outbursts up to the age of 12, when my family escaped as refugees from Moldova, my country of birth. Then, I suddenly transitioned from being a very unruly child, to a very calm—even *too* calm—one. The new environment affected me in such a way that the psychic energy I had been manifesting outwardly all those years was suddenly internalized. The culture shock inhibited me to the point that I lost the desire to socialize and go to school. Because that in itself was not a good-enough reason, I tried to magnify my inner discomfort to convince my parents that my stomach really *did* hurt.

My parents didn't believe me initially, so I had to utilize all my creative energy in order to appear sick. After a while of continuous attempts, there was no longer a need to pretend—the pain became very real. My parents still didn't believe me, though, since I'd cried wolf too many times. However, they were concerned enough to send me for various medical checkups, just in case. For about a year, I went through a series of tests until, finally, the doctors diagnosed my illness.

The day I was given a prognosis of the terminal illness was not a sad one for me. On the contrary, I was overjoyed that my parents finally believed me. It sealed my faith that suffering could be a way to deserve, and attain, loving attention.

Love beyond the Fairy Tale

Don Sinchi listened to me as I shared my insights with him. He said, "Creating either a fully positive or negative imprint in the river of consciousness is as elaborate as building an irrigation channel. You have to wish for the river to change course first, by determining a new route. Second, you must work on a construction plan. Third, you have to fulfill your plan through a lot of effort. Finally, you must feel satisfied with the end result."

Reflecting on these four factors, I could now see how my suffering had been birthed from my own ignorance—from wishing to be ill, just to have my parents care for me . . . even though I hadn't known any better. Then, I planned for it, worked hard to make the illness real, and was happy with the consequences. Having the genetic predisposition for that specific illness, of course, also helped crystallize the disease in my body.

I told the elder how the wave of remembrance practice took me to my memory of my parents' conflict and separation. I saw it as the initial trauma that changed the route of my consciousness stream toward illness and impacted all the intimate relationships in my life. One of the most challenging parts of the practice involved the recollection of my first great love marrying my best friend. No matter how much I tried to forget, the connection between my inner and outer universe kept pointing me to the inner source where suffering originated.

I was so disillusioned by the relationship with my first love that I emigrated once again—this time to the United States, with my family, at the age of 19. My family settled in a New York suburb, where I felt lonelier than ever in the midst of a huge metropolis bustling with people. I had no connection to a spiritual practice or any knowledge of holistic medicine—and I was going through a culture shock once again, but this time alongside severe depression. It was that experience of being completely lost that served as an initial invitation to embark on the path of self-realization and natural healing.

Remembering the discord between my parents and my own broken heart, I asked Don Sinchi about the higher meaning of intimate relationships in his culture.

Don Sinchi laughed and said: "It's a very large topic; there's a whole branch of Evolutionary Science dedicated to it in the Amazon, called *Pusanga*. Nowadays, it's mostly known as love magic, accomplished with the help of perfumed spells and icaros that engage the raw powers of attraction. However, even though instinctual energies appear to be very powerful, they are neither lasting nor reliable. The good Pusangeros will tell you that even the best spells are temporary—and if there is no conscious evolutionary connection for true love to manifest, then the spell will eventually fade. True love becomes a reality only when you begin to be true to yourself by facing your shadows and igniting your heart's spark over and over again."

According to Don Sinchi, Pusanga was meant as another reminder to transform passion into compassion by awakening the higher wisdom of our sexual energy. Unconsciously grasping on to their appearances without seeing their symbolic meaning on the inner level is disastrous. For example, imagine that you meet a person you are extremely attracted to. You feel a tremendous amount of passion that connects you to your creative spark when you are around this person. But the relationship goes south, and you're devastated. You feel hurt, betrayed, and lost—because you mistakenly believe that the amazing emotions you experienced were caused by your lover. You fail to see that what was awakened was your own potential, and the person was a catalyst rather than the source. What you were drawn to were the deep inner qualities essential to all humans, which your lover's external appearance and behavior reminded you of.

This approach is like trying to get closer to the sun by jumping into every swampy puddle that merely reflects the light but can never be the source of it.

"Toé, with its intoxicating scent, is a master plant of the highest degree within the Pusanga mystery school, because it works with underground water streams," Don Sinchi explained. "After a prolonged training, initiation, and preparation, the Mother of Toé can help you navigate the darkness of the underworld. It's up to each practitioner, however, to establish a genuine incentive for the creative energy to be liberated from its vicious cycles into the light of heart-centered awareness. To develop the motivation necessary to ingest this sacred plant, one must first dive into the muddy puddles enough times to realize that the source of light is found in the opposite direction."

Don Sinchi went on to explain that in ancient times, the focus of the intimate relationship was for two people to look in the same direction together, rather than obsess over each other. The evolutionary path of the heart was about mutual support and inspiration, not the suffocating dependency on external conditions and appearances.

I thought about the way relationships in modern society typically went. I told Don Sinchi that, from all I'd witnessed, obsession and infatuation ran rampant, and global divorce rates were the highest they'd ever been.

My personal experience of intimate relationships was that people tend to project their idea of the perfect partner onto another human who serves as the perfect screen. It's the prince on the white horse, or the princess in the tower, reenacting an ancient archetypal spectacle. It seems to start with some kind of fairy-tale fantasy in which everyone is destined to live happily ever after. Usually, this phase lasts around six months. At a certain point, however, a plot twist develops. Instead of seeing the significant other as a human being, we think, "No, you have to be that princess or that prince for me! I need you to be a certain way for me because that keeps the play going!" The other person can't keep up with their role, which upsets us, because waking up from the fairy tale is too painful. The fairy tale ends, and the soap opera begins!

Don Sinchi chuckled when I shared all this with him. Sympathetically, he offered, "By becoming fluent in the dream language of nature, the intimate relationship becomes an invitation to cultivate the attractive qualities that the significant other is reflecting in you. You must also be ready to face the shadows of your ignorance—this is another cornerstone of a healthy relationship. But if you conveniently forget to face yourself and expect someone else to do all the work for you, the relationship degrades. When intimacy is based on projections and expectations, it becomes draining. Sooner or later, such a relationship becomes a shadow version of itself—the prince on the white horse becomes the troll under the bridge, and the princess in the tower becomes a malevolent hag. All the inner shadows in any long-term relationship eventually rise to the surface. Yet, if people don't wish to face themselves, they blame their shadows on the other person."

He explained the purpose of the evolutionary relationship, which is to share freedom with one another. You wish for yourself and your lover to be human beings first and foremost. An evolutionary foundation of relatedness and friendship allows for the most fulfilling relationship to blossom. There has to be mutual encouragement for each person to do their own inner work. Instinctual infatuation can never provide such a foundation, although, of course, biological attraction is also essential. There has to be a basic attraction, but it also needs to transcend itself so that a solid friendship—based on a deep affinity and connection to heart-centered life values—can develop. The true glue of any sustainable relationship is the willingness to walk alongside each other on the path of awakening the heart's wisdom, through thick and thin.

"Without a deeper friendship, it's a recipe for disaster," Don Sinchi said. "The initial connection is not sustainable at all! Inevitably, the moment of truth arrives: 'I'm here with this person—what do we have in common besides our inevitably waning animalistic attraction?' The differences in life values will become more apparent over time, until they're either faced or make the relationship fall apart. That's why a foundation of friendship is so instrumental, so each individual can keep blooming over time, just like these Toé flowers. With a steady root foundation, the wish-fulfilling tree of an inspiring relationship can develop for the benefit of the entire ecosystem."

Don Sinchi paused to observe a hummingbird fly over to drink the nectar of the flowers in front of us. Then he looked back at me and continued, "This brings us back to our Amazonian cosmology of how human beings are meant to be happy, just like birds fly in the sky. Of course, we can dream about the divine union that leads us into timeless joy, but without understanding the inner language of evolution, we will be duped by appearances. By awakening the longing for inner wholeness, however, you can be nurtured by the nectar of all those essential human qualities you find so irresistibly attractive in others. If you keep expecting others to always do it for you, however, you end up hurting them."

Don Sinchi explained that when we cultivate these qualities, we face all our shadows with the motivation to dedicate our blossoming heart to the well-being of others. We become the cross-pollinating hummingbirds, who drink the nectar of wisdom from the flowers of collective experience. Divine union is based on complementary opposites. We are unconsciously drawn to the polar opposites in our life because opposites attract. If it is Father Sun's qualities a person is attracted to, then maybe that means they are more intuitive, receptive, and emotional, and the conceptual approach to life is irresistibly attractive to them, albeit confusing! If someone finds Mother Earth's qualities seductive, perhaps they are drawn to an emotional, fluid, and spontaneous way of being, which is typically incomprehensible to an overdeveloped logical mind. There are many qualities of the divine union expressed through various life-forms and natural elements—and we can learn from all of them.

"We may even find ourselves pulled by different qualities at different times in our lives, based on what is needed for us to open up in each phase of the evolutionary journey. By uniting the mind and the heart within, you begin to witness the wholeness of the greater organism in each moment," Don Sinchi said.

The elder took a pause and blew the mapacho smoke in the direction of the Toé's roots.

I asked, "How does the divine union you just described apply to my life? Personally, I have experienced nothing like it, either in my parents or in any of my intimate relationships."

The elder looked at me. "Because you are a reluctant hero on an evolutionary path, everything that happened to you thus far has been a continuous wake-up call. You were shown all the ways of being that are unfulfilling to your heart, which is what you share about the world you come from, where inner wholeness is not the conscious focus of life. Unconsciously grasping at the appearances that merely symbolize your inner transformation, you end up more miserable, lost, and confused than ever. The Great Spirit of Mother Nature has been intentionally guiding you all along. It's the same message that is coming through more and more clearly as you progress on the path of remembrance.

"The difference in how intimate relationships are experienced in mainstream society versus ancient times goes further still. Today, intimate relationships are mostly about, 'I met this person, and we're going to create a wall around us to experience intimacy, vulnerability, and tenderness, but only inside our little bubble that's closed off from the rest of the world.' Whereas the ancient perspective of marriage was for it to become the beacon of awakening unconditional love to infinity and beyond.

"In the Amazonian cosmovision, Mother Earth and Father Sun symbolize the union of consciousness and love being expressed by myriad life-forms in the universe. Each life-form represents the unique qualities of Noble Masculine and Divine Feminine, which allow wholeness to be alchemized within. In many ancient cultures, the deep love people have for each other is dedicated to the benefit of all beings. The relationship must radiate outward, rather than collapse onto itself. That is the natural progression of the evolutionary journey."

Tool: Understanding Intimate Relationships

Many emotional blockages and unresolved tensions are formed through the sequence of our past intimate relationships. Apply the wave of remembrance practice to all your past lovers, with the recognition of the initial "honeymoon" phase as the anchor for positive memories that each person was ultimately guiding you toward. Next, travel through the "eclipse" phase, full of challenges and painful lessons, that was pointing you toward the path of your evolutionary journey. In what ways was each partner helping you return to freedom and wholeness? We all have unique lessons to learn, so see whether you can find similar patterns across different relationships.

The Wave of Dreaming

I must have looked like a deer in the headlights, struggling to comprehend a totally new perspective about relationships. Don Sinchi noticed my puzzled expression and lit his pipe, blowing the smoke all over me and the Toé tree until all of us, the tree included, were enveloped in a large cloud.

After the smoke dissipated, he smiled. "Don't worry, I can relate to how you feel because I was in the same place myself once upon a time. It will make more sense to you as you progress along this path. The truth is way too simple for our complicated minds to understand. For now, simply remember not to seek love outside of yourself to compensate for the lack thereof within, but be inspired by all your relationships to nurture whatever tiny seeds and sprouts of essential humanity you can find inside. Easier said than done, of course, but it all starts with admitting to yourself when you are not doing it."

Don Sinchi announced that he would now introduce me more deeply to the dreaming wave so that I could master the boundless love that went beyond appearances.

"Oh, I almost forgot—remember to place a Toé flower under your pillow every night for better results, as it will help awaken your capacity for dreaming vividly," Don Sinchi said. "Now, I will demonstrate to you how to ask this plant spirit for its flowers."

Don Sinchi asked permission from the Toé plant by placing a handful of loose mapacho at its roots as he stood in silent prayer for a minute. I noticed that the elder chose the tree that emanated the most beautiful smell and had the most flowers. He carefully removed one yellow flower with red tips and handed it to me. We then headed back and called it a night. I diligently followed Don Sinchi's dreaming instructions from that night on.

A few days later, he came to visit me in my hut in the late afternoon and asked how my healing journey had been thus far. I told him how grateful I was to him for reminding me of our essential human nature and the healing power of the heart to forgive and accept. I could further see that there was a higher purpose to all my misfortunes. As a result, I began experiencing tremendous peace and a sense of relief engulfing my entire being. The inner peace, in turn, provided me with greater clarity and deeper insights into my evolutionary journey.

Don Sinchi listened to me while packing his pipe with fresh mapacho. When I finished sharing, he lit his pipe and took a few long puffs. "This is where the dreaming wave can be beneficial— by helping you recognize where the life energy within you can flow in greater harmony with your original evolutionary imprint. The ancient ones were in constant communication with the Great Spirit of the rainforest through their dreams. As I shared with you before, the Great Spirit communicates in a language that is mostly forgotten in our day and age. In order to reestablish an intentional relationship with the spirit of our Great Mother, we study her peculiar language."

He told me that modern language is full of mental concepts and overintellectualization. In a false hierarchy, reason is placed above the heart. The language of the ancestors, on the other hand, is much more related to the language of nature and the wisdom of the heart. Mythical heroic journeys, legendary symbols, metaphors, and parables are the primary attributes of Mother Nature's communication. Nature continuously emphasizes our higher evolutionary purpose as a priority in the mundane hamster wheel of survival. The language of Mother Nature mirrors her indestructible spirit of interconnected intelligence.

When the original Evolutionary Science became fragmented, it was the Achuar tribe that preserved the specific lineage of working consciously with dreams. "I myself have integrated this practice from my Achuar elder friends. In our recent conversations, Romancito, I spoke of how everything we are dreaming of is manifesting from our true nature. We are always in tune with the consciousness of the Great Spirit. Our dreams directly communicate to us how to remember the primordial, ocean-like nature of who we are. The wave of remembrance practice teaches us how to unravel major knots of emotional tension in our lives. The practice of the dreaming wave is a more advanced one and provides us with a detailed energetic blueprint for evolution. It specifically points out black holes in our luminous energy bodies, where the light of consciousness is called to bring a much-needed resolution. The cultivation of essential qualities and profound human values is instrumental for our individual existence to merge with the universal ocean of all-abiding presence."

Hearing the elder mention the mysterious ocean of the Great Spirit before had made me think of the collective unconscious, also referred to as the superconscious in Jungian psychology. I mentioned this to Don Sinchi, whose face lit up.

"To become superconscious, you must open your heart to all that life has to offer. A heroic journey into the underworld is required before accessing the treasury of human potential. Shadow work is an essential foundation to clear all your personal baggage that stands in the way of your limitless nature. You must learn how to channel the most basic survival impulses of the human organism through the many stages of your evolution. Only then can life heal at the core. The dreaming wave is an effective tool for such a purpose."

Don Sinchi informed me that the first step in the dreaming wave was to write down whatever one remembered from their dreams at night first thing in the morning, so that was where I would begin.

"But I often do not have any dreams or end up remembering only meaningless fragments," I insisted.

Don Sinchi responded patiently while puffing on his pipe: "Even if you wake up and you don't remember a thing, you should try to write down at least a vague sense of what is left over from the night. Initially, it's enough to note the mood you wake up in the morning with. The reason for writing is to let your dream body know that your dreams matter to you. Conscious pathways then begin to develop for you to hear the communication of your higher self, which is the wisdom of the entire organism that your ego is just now getting to know."

I wondered aloud why it was so difficult for me to remember my dreams or to even feel that I was having any.

"The primary focus of modern society does not include the more 'ethereal' aspects of life," Don Sinchi said. "Dreams are just not that important for modern living—and if we don't focus on something, it becomes a lesser priority. Because the awareness in our life is limited by the degree of our maturity, there's only so much of it to go around. Who cares about a dreamy evolution when everyone is preoccupied only with material existence? We are all affected by the collective state of humanity in one way or another, which is why we have to retrain ourselves to bring all the facets of our greater whole into everyday awareness."

Don Sinchi went on to explain that once I'd developed a discipline of recording my dreams every morning upon waking up, I would start remembering them with greater clarity. At a certain point, my consciousness would home in to such an extent that I would remember many dreams every night in the most vivid detail.

"I will periodically review your accumulated dream logs with you so that you can learn the evolutionary language of universal patterns that lead to higher consciousness," said Don Sinchi.

"Is there something specific I should be watching out for, Don Sinchi?"

"Well, you should always approach this practice from the perspective that everything in your dream is a facet of you. The background, landscapes in which the dream occurs, objects, situations, and people are all different representations of the greater you. That's why it's helpful to try to remember every detail of your dreams at night to begin seeing the dreamlike nature of everyday life as well. All people and situations in life are symbols and metaphors. Every speck of dust has profound meaning."

With that guidance, the Rimyurá sent me back into my hut to explore the inner landscapes of Nature, reflected so magnificently in the rainforest all around us.

The Dreamer's Responsibility

I had been diligent with the wave of remembrance practice, as well as the Huayra-Otorongo breath; now, I began to engage with the dreaming wave in earnest. I developed a ritual of intention setting every night per Don Sinchi's instructions; this involved asking permission from the Toé plant by the creek nearby, explaining to it why I needed its flower, and then placing it under my pillow before going to sleep.

After a few nights, I began to feel inebriated by the fragrance of the flower to the point where I'd have visions even before falling asleep. The first signs of progress appeared within the first few days. Although I was still unable to remember the content of my dreams, I started to recall that, at the very least, I was having them.

Frustrated, I went to Don Sinchi to ask for guidance. He listened to my account and responded, "Remember, Romancito, that dreams are communications from a superconscious being, speaking to you in the language of your own life experience. You can only understand what the higher consciousness is saying to you based on the context of *your* life. A dream dictionary can never substitute self-discovery. There is, however, a way to map the landmarks of your inner landscape by recognizing the building blocks of all life in the universe. Our people refer to them as the autonomous spirits of Mother Nature that are all linked by the Great Spirit through our own personality traits. They are the threads from which the fabric of reality is woven, embedded at the core of our being. This is how divine union occurs. Without the union of complementary opposites in Nature, none of us would be born and life would not be sustained on this planet."

"Don Sinchi, throughout our time together you have been using alternating terms like Mother Earth, Father Sun, Mother Nature, the Great Spirit, Universal Consciousness, Unconditional Love, and so on. I've been intuitively interpreting them as being interchangeable. Is this correct?"

"Before I answer your question, you must know that a good scout of the inner landscape must be ready to retrace their steps and get real with himself. Some are too stubborn and arrogant to admit when they're lost, so they get even more lost as time goes by. Once you acknowledge that you are lost, the journey to find yourself begins. Until then, you will neither be humble nor receptive enough for the dedication to find your way home to be genuine. That is the foundation of our friendship: to love the truth more than each other's personalities. You recognize the spark of dedication to the truth in me, and vice versa. As a fellow truth seeker, you can ask any sincere question without being embarrassed. Without that kind of friendship, the evolutionary path is meaningless."

The elder squinted his eyes, evaluating my demeanor.

I responded, "I chose to stay here with you, Don Sinchi, because I recognize that same spark in you that I have in myself, but in you it's much brighter. Although your guidance has been instrumental for me thus far, it's your dedication to the truth of being that I find the most essential in my healing journey. I don't mind being reprimanded or even insulted by you because I know we're both dedicated to freedom from suffering and ignorance. I care about learning more than I care how ridiculous I look when asking stupid questions."

Don Sinchi continued to evaluate me, this time with his signature mischievous smile. "I am happy that we are on the same page, Romancito. This time, however, I am not going to reprimand you, because you're right—the terms I have been using *are* interchangeable."

He explained that the majestic spirits of Nature were represented by symbols because their essence is beyond form. The many facets of the divine union were expressed through an infinitely diverse variety of appearances, both in this material existence and in our inner worlds.

The Great Mother, as the ultimate expression of the feminine, represents the unconditional love that is always available to everyone, without the need to earn or be worthy of it. The Great Father is the impartial light of consciousness that perpetually realizes the greater depths of her boundless love. Although the Great Mother's womb is pregnant with limitless possibilities, without the impartial, brilliant light of consciousness that is the Great Father, evolution would not gather momentum.

Our inner qualities that support the profound values of the shared heart are also the enlightened aspects of Mother Nature. It is through these essential qualities that she births all life-forms. Everything and everyone in our lives are metaphors that serve to point out the diverse qualities of complementary universal opposites. The trees, the rivers, the sky, the earth, the mountains and valleys, the body and spirit, the mind and the heart—these are all expressions of the complementary opposites in Nature. Yet, as Don Sinchi explained, it is up to each of us to connect the dots between the universal qualities that this collective dream called reality is continuously reflecting to us. In other words, we need to avoid being fooled by appearances and to remember that every form that exists is here for the purpose of leading us back to a higher consciousness.

"I have already mentioned to you once how the ancestors personified Goddess Nature, remember?" inquired Don Sinchi. "Each human is familiar with at least the most basic expressions of love and kindness, as well as the opposite, and can recognize them without words in oneself and others. They are qualities that we either strive for or inhibit in ourselves, out of fear or mistrust. The light of your highest potential and the shadows of your emotional knots are all interwoven in your being. The totality of these qualities is also expressed through all the interactions in our dreams. Dreams are communications of the Great Spirit, which always encourages the healthy balance of complementary opposites within us."

I felt that everything I'd learned from Don Sinchi could be correlated with the universal motifs documented by transpersonal psychology across cultures the world over. I was, however, still at my wit's end about connecting the dots between my dreams, my life, and my feelings and emotions. I asked Don Sinchi how I could learn to decipher the messages of the Great Spirit in my dreams.

"The language of Nature is based on intuitive associations," he said. "It takes time for the conceptual mind to refrain from interpreting dream content literally, as meaningless impressions unrelated to self-realization. The presence of an experienced guide is beneficial to illuminate the way in the initially obscure realm of the intuition. In fact, that is the purpose of the teacher in our tradition—the maestro is like the moon, illuminating your path through the rainforest at night. Don't try to get to the moon by blindly worshiping the teacher. Only when you can find your way through the dark forest of your ignorance, guided by the moonlight, will you truly honor the teacher."

Don Sinchi got up and encouragingly patted me on my shoulder. He then looked out of my hut at the moonlit forest. "This is my time now to be guided by Mother Moon to my home." He winked at me and left.

I thought of what Don Sinchi had said. I was familiar with dream dictionaries, which seemed to turn the task of interpreting one's nighttime visions into a fun, sometimes inspiring, but often superficial game. But according to the elder, it went much deeper than that. Understanding my personal dream language entailed taking full responsibility for my life.

I went to ask the nearby Toé tree for its flower. I felt grateful that it had taken me getting so lost in life to embark on the journey of finding my true self.

Tool: Mapping the Inner Landscape of Dreams

You can engage the dreaming wave practice with other flowers, such as lavender, the smell of which is also known to induce restful sleep, or even essential oils in your preferred scent. Before going to bed at night, spend at least an hour without any electronics; right before falling asleep, make a clear intention to remember your dreams. As you record your dreams, begin to chart the map of your inner landscapes by noticing any prevalent themes that come up in your dreams. Every aspect of your dream experiences—such as the time of day, location (city or natural landscape), as well as people and objects that are present—can be traced back to the complementary opposites of life that the Indigenous people refer to as the feminine and masculine qualities. Over time, you'll begin to recognize the unique dance between these complementary opposites within you, as you find equilibrium between the mind and the heart.

REFLECTIONS

- So often in our modern world, love is based on a dance of superficial appearances: looks, status, wealth, and even shared interests can serve to distract us from the deeper gift of love—a mutual evolutionary journey that ideally helps us connect with a higher consciousness and dedicate ourselves to the well-being of all, rather than getting caught up in our own fairy tale. *In what ways have your intimate relationships diminished or amplified your higher potential? How did the extent to which you were caught up in the modern drama of "love" impact your and your partners' happiness and well-being?*

- Life is a dance of complementary opposites—and without this union of complementary opposites in Nature, none of us would be born and life could not be sustained on this planet. *Consider the complementary opposites that exist in both your inner and outer worlds. In what ways do they coalesce to create a greater sense of aliveness and awaken your own essential nature? What do you think contributes to a greater sense of harmony between opposites, versus conflict between opposites?*

- Don Sinchi helped me understand that dreams are not just visions caused by randomly firing neurons while we sleep; they are powerful communications from a super-conscious being, speaking to us in the language of our own life experience. We can only understand what the higher consciousness is saying to us based on the context of our life, and a dream dictionary can never be a stand-in for our self-discovery. *Think of the last dream you had, as well as its most powerful symbols. Based on your life today, what do you think the Great Spirit was attempting to communicate to you?*

CHAPTER 12

THE PRACTICAL NATURE OF DREAMS

Within a week of the last conversation with Don Sinchi, I began recollecting brief events accompanied by feelings in my dreams. What proved to be the most helpful in my healing process was the point when meaningful encounters with different characters in my dreams began to emerge in my post-dream introspection.

Don Sinchi explained to me that besides the "small" dreams, which can shed light on the process of transformation, there are also "big" dreams. The big dreams are distinguished by their vivid and memorable qualities. They can leave a powerful impression on one's life. These are the dreams to watch out for, because they mark pivotal thresholds in one's remembrance journey and can be consciously engaged as evolutionary rites of passage.

The first big dream occurred for me shortly after that conversation with the Yahua elder. In the dream, I initially found myself on a large cruise liner in the middle of the sea. The cruise ship was also a city, where I lived alongside my parents and friends. One day, I decided to leave that ship and travel to the Amazon rainforest.

I had gotten myself a little motorboat that could also function as a pedal boat in case of emergency. Shortly after departing, I ran out of fuel and had to start pedaling the rest of the way. After a prolonged effort, I found an entrance to the Amazon River. Continuing to pedal upriver, I finally docked on the shore. As soon as my boat touched the riverbank, it transformed into a big mechanical bear, like in the *Transformers* cartoons I watched as a child. I began riding the bear, following a trail that ran deep into the rainforest.

After galloping through the rainforest on the mechanical bear for a while, I encountered a tremendous black she-wolf that jumped out from the bushes, right in front of the bear. Although my bear was big, he seemed small and weak compared to the she-wolf. At the sight of the she-wolf, the bear whimpered, dropped me on the ground, and ran into the bushes.

I landed in the mud, face down, before the she-wolf. Lying there at the mercy of the wild beast, I felt no fear. Strangely enough, I was at ease with my vulnerability. The she-wolf approached me, sniffing. She carefully picked me up with her teeth, latching on to the skin at the back of my neck, and carried me into the rainforest as if I were one of her runaway pups.

I woke up exhilarated and refreshed. Quickly recording my dream, I went to see Don Sinchi. Upon hearing my dream, his face lit up. He informed me that I'd just had one of those big dreams he'd told me to watch out for, and that it was an excellent sign from the Great Spirit, indicating my progress on the healing path.

Closing his eyes, the elder took a few moments to contemplate before finally speaking. "I'd like to first remind you that the way we work with dreams is by not taking their messages literally. Everything has a higher meaning, pointing to your evolutionary journey of awakening."

He went on to tell me that the large cruise ship in my dream represented my life in society. Both my parents were there, as their conflict and the trauma it had caused me had been the catalyst for my healing journey. I had taken my wounding along with me onto the mothership of society, which was leisurely cruising through the ocean of daily commotion. As a conforming member of society, my life lacked the true freedom to be myself, which caused suffering. It was essential to discover for myself what this life was all about, beyond the familiar tourist traps of generic attractions and superficial values. Before embarking on my healing journey to the Amazon, my earthly parents and the rest of society had been responsible for my choices in life—that is, I was either following what I'd been told or rebelling against it. To honor the calling of my heart, I had to abandon my infantile state and make conscious decisions in service of my awakening.

Don Sinchi explained that the small boat I'd traveled on signified an exodus from social norms. My quest led me upriver, against the stream of conformity and back to the origins of human civilization at the heart of Mother Nature. The limited amount of fuel represented my initial motivation, stemming from a realization that conditioned existence was not aligned with my spirit. The wilderness of the Amazon rainforest represented my decision to return to a natural, uninhibited state. The fuel running out and the need to pedal pointed to the need for perspiration to replace the inspiration on the path of self-realization—that is, I had to make an immense effort on the path to truly appreciate its efficacy in transforming the unruly monkey mind and its lifelong habits.

Once I'd made it to the shore of the Amazon, the boat turned into a mechanical bear. Both the boat and the bear were one and the same and pointed out the different practices and spiritual techniques I'd acquired on my path so far. These techniques, however, were artificial and inefficient, even though they'd served a purpose. Once I arrived in the abode of my true nature, these conceptual methods could not carry me. That's when I encountered the black mother wolf, a powerful manifestation of Nature and a symbol of my deep intuitive connection to the life force within me. I was currently replacing the robotic methods with an intuitive approach. The wolf was a symbol of my individual evolutionary journey—honoring the wisdom of the ancestors and howling at the moonlight that guided the way home. Her pitch blackness meant that, for a long time, she was my shadow. I had repressed the wild force of creativity within me to the point of self-harm. My personality was now being taught by Spirit to respect Nature inside out, by being humble and fearlessly loving. The Mother of my autoimmune disease had brought my conceptual mind here, so it could surrender to the wisdom of fierce unconditional love.

Don Sinchi gently smiled and said, "You have been gestating in the dark womb of conditioned existence throughout your entire life, until now. The she-wolf picked you up, as if you were one of her lost cubs, which signifies a rebirth into your higher purpose. Adopted by the wild, you no longer belong to the society you came from. You are now learning what it means to be a free-spirited child of this mysterious universe."

Balancing the Feminine and Masculine

I marveled at Don Sinchi's ability to so clearly bring the symbols of my dream into greater clarity. "It all makes perfect sense, Don Sinchi," I said. "Spirit is encouraging me to remember the nature of interconnectedness that awakens the heart's wisdom."

Don Sinchi nodded, satisfied with my response. "Now that you understand the importance of hearing the communication of your higher self, your dreams should become even more vivid. Keep watching out for the big ones—you will get another soon enough."

A few days later, I had another one of the big dreams that Don Sinchi had said I would. In the dream, I was a beautiful woman. I had never had a dream in which I was a woman, but it felt surprisingly natural to me. I was naked and chained in a gully of a big sailboat voyaging across the ocean. I was being kept prisoner by the captain of the ship, who was a crude seafarer. After many years of being stranded in the ocean, the sailboat finally arrived at a tropical island. The captain came into the gully and unchained me, and we went up to the main deck together. He escorted me into a big, beautiful mansion, located on the island, and left me by myself in a sunny corridor by the entrance, while he went upstairs. I stood there, not knowing what to do with my newfound freedom, when a child emerged from one of the doors.

He was an innocent, lovely child, maybe about three or four years old. He approached me and appeared to deeply trust me. I looked at the child, still grappling with all the years of abuse I had sustained as a naked woman chained in the gully of the ship. I sensed the captain was related to the child. Thoughts of taking revenge on the captain by punishing the child coursed through my head. Suddenly, I awoke drenched in cold sweat, deeply shaken by the intensity and realness of my dream. It felt like I had lived an entire lifetime in one night.

I got up and took a morning dunk in the creek on the way to see Don Sinchi. Eventually, I found him in the medicine kitchen, preparing another batch of Ayahuasca. He invited me to join him and, noticing my distress, asked me to share what had happened.

After I finished relating my dream, the elder sat for a while, gazing into the bubbling cauldron. Then, without lifting his eyes from the cauldron, he began to share his interpretation of my dream.

According to Don Sinchi, the sailboat, just like in my previous dream, represented the wandering of my personality through the ocean of the Great Spirit in a desperate quest for liberation. The ocean was vast and easy to get lost in. The naked woman represented me—or, more precisely, my intuitive connection to the creative source within. The feminine, creative part of me was finally emerging after being repressed for so many years. I had created my own chains of conditioning as a response to the unfavorable emotional winds that brought about the painful circumstances of my life. The captain was none other than the crudeness of my personality, which was overprotective of the inner child—who'd given him the power to roam the high seas in the first place.

It was time to consciously honor and uplift my feminine side in order for my creative energy to channel healing rather than self-destruction. After all, the child in the dream was my own innocence, which was also finally emerging to be healed through all my practices of anchoring in compassion, forgiveness, and empathy.

The memory of the conflict between my parents, with me entangled in the midst of it, suddenly became so vivid that my body was instantly covered in cold sweat. I took it as a sign to share my deeper process with the elder.

"Don Sinchi, through the wave of remembrance, I've been reliving the traumatic events of my childhood. Because of my parents' conflict, I suppressed my creative feminine side, while using the masculine as a way to tough it out through life's storms. How can I balance my inner masculine and feminine nature for the childlike spark to be fully supported?"

"You made yourself a promise long ago to never act like your father, while lacking trust in your mother at the same time. You know, Romancito, you will never become a real man if you cannot embrace your inner woman! Only through the harmonious balance of the masculine and feminine can your childlike nature awaken to the evolutionary path!"

I felt an energetic knot being dissolved in my belly. Like pieces of the puzzle, all the work I had been doing in the ceremonies, dietas, and the wave practices began to culminate in ripples of blissful realization.

Don Sinchi told me that although I could now see the core issues that had been responsible for my conditioning in the first place, this was just the beginning. "From here on, it's up to you to engage with all the wave practices to keep realizing how the traumatic imprints from your childhood affected you in the later years of your life all the way up to now. Only when you surrender all the trapped tensions that are still remaining in you, and give them back to the ocean of your heart, will you be totally free."

"What will happen to me once I do that?"

He responded nonchalantly, "Nothing special, except that you will continue your evolutionary healing journey, step by step, toward the infinite potential seeded in you by the Great Spirit upon birth. The Ashuar people, who initiated me into the dreaming wave, are known as the best scouts and warriors of the rainforest. However, it's not physical strength that gives them such prowess and resilience. What gives them advantage over others is how well they are versed in the language of Nature. Seeing through appearances allows the Ashuars to embrace pure innocence as their highest purpose. Once innocence can stand up for itself, no longer afraid of getting lost, the exploration and mapping of our inner wilderness begins."

He could see my puzzlement, at which point he assured me that it would become clear to me through experience, because words could not do it justice. For now, I would continue using the tools and applying them skillfully to life's predicaments.

"Remember that it's not about fixing the past, but making sure that the unresolved emotional charges of your past are not messing with you in the present. In Evolutionary Science, our emotional traumas are known as sacred guardians. They diligently safeguard the emanations of the Great Spirit trapped inside us by our fear of the unknown. Your most essential healing is the healing of your relationship with constant, inevitable change."

Don Sinchi told me that each of us has a choice in life: On one hand, we could be haunted by change, while resisting our circumstances and trying to maintain a fixed identity filled with soul-draining stories. On the other hand, we could abide in the heart's unwavering wisdom, which welcomes change as nourishment from the Great Mother. Change only serves to remind us that the unconditional love our hearts are capable of sustaining is exponential and never-ending. Only the boundless wisdom of the heart is capable of witnessing constant change and remaining steadfast, like the eye in the center of a storm.

"In case you are still struggling, like myself and my predecessors were at your stage of the healing journey, Romancito, I have something to further assist your heroic baby steps," Don Sinchi said. "Your healing is beginning to resonate with the frequency of the rainforest. At this stage of your initiation into Evolutionary Science, other master plant teachers that are on par with Ayahuasca can be introduced. During these dietas, you will stay in another, more isolated hut, deeper in the rainforest, for prolonged periods of time. You are not to speak with anyone except me and whomever I authorize. You will still be allowed, however, to partake in ceremonies with me and my colleagues, students, and patients."

I thanked Don Sinchi and went back to my hut. I had never been so open with anyone in my life, nor had I felt so seen—without the fear of being judged or misunderstood. I understood that he was a clear mirror for me to realize my own mirrorlike nature. The mirror doesn't break when it reflects something ugly and doesn't bend out of shape when it reflects something beautiful.

I was beginning to drop my armor of stale concepts and ideas that had guarded my heart for so long. The Yahua elder, with gentle firmness, was simply helping me usher in my own potential. He was neither my savior nor my parent, but a dear friend in whom I could recognize my own truth.

I felt immense gratitude for Don Sinchi, the moon illuminating the path through my enchanted inner forest. That night, I closed my eyes and surrendered to the dream realm of infinite mystery. The healing journey was just beginning, and I now had the essential foundation to coherently answer the call of the Great Spirit.

Tool: Connecting the Dots between Masculine and Feminine

The masculine and feminine are inseparable within us. The ocean can be simultaneously turbulent on the surface and calm in its depth, just as the rainforest is loving and ferocious at the same time. As Evolutionary Science guides us to see beyond appearances, the dance of inner qualities guides us toward inner wholeness and equilibrium.

One way to relate to the healthy balance between the masculine and feminine is to develop our ability to be brave enough to be vulnerable. Instead of using your creative energy to pretend to be strong or avoid your issues, you can be vulnerable from a place of empowerment—and, without any drama, engage your creative energy to face life's predicaments with childlike ingenuity.

Here is a creative approach to connect the dots between masculine and feminine within your own life more profoundly: Draw or paint your weaknesses, challenges, and adversity using images that represent them for you. Now, draw all the inspirations, passions, and uplifting qualities using different images. Next, find a connecting link between the two—just like the Taoist symbols of yin and yang, with the learning curve between the two and the essence of each one found within the center of the other. You can also make a circle around all your images because the circle represents wholeness within the Amazonian tradition. You can engage this practice in a similar way with music, dance, poems, sculpting, etc. The main focus is to make the creative process relevant to your immediate challenges and inspirations.

Back to Wholeness

Throughout the first six months of my evolutionary healing process in the Amazon, I witnessed many miraculous healings among the local villagers. Some were even brought to the ceremonies on the brink of death. Seeing their transformation greatly reaffirmed and strengthened my trust in the Indigenous medicine and the Evolutionary Science tradition.

My physical and emotional health continuously improved after each ceremony, but as Don Sinchi had foretold, this was only the beginning; the cost of entry was a relentless battle with my inner demons. Luckily, I understood by now that the demons were not some phantasmagorical creatures, but my own fears, inhibitions, repressed emotions, and dramas from the past, which had all become concretized as habitual patterns.

Utilizing the powerful tools of transformation that Don Sinchi generously shared with me allowed me some potent glimpses into the radiance inherent in all beings. Free from the encumbrances of concepts like "good" and "bad," I could connect both the animalistic and the divine aspects of my life together. With the help of ceremonial transmissions, I reached a threshold that allowed me to clearly see how I'd inadvertently activated a genetic predisposition to my terminal illness as a small child. With the guidance of Don Sinchi and the spiritual discipline that accompanied the sacred plant ceremonies, I began to take full responsibility for all my past actions, decisions, and wishes. Ignorance was no longer an excuse I could use to keep running from the unresolved issues that had haunted me throughout my life.

By reversing my habitual patterns, I began to see the psychosomatic source of my sickness. The root of my suffering had to do with my reactive behavior and not the circumstances of my life, difficult as they were.

My time with the elder had taught me something I still carry with me to this day: habitual patterns of conditioned behavior get deeply ingrained in the mind through spiritual amnesia. Therefore, the living wisdom of the ancestors engages the evolutionary path with a great deal of repetition. The same essence of being must be introduced through many angles. We bring the bird's-eye view into all the facets of our lives, from peak experiences to the most mundane events. When our five earthly senses are brought into unwavering, openhearted presence, the sixth celestial sense is born. Each moment then becomes a profound catalyst for evolution.

Our evolutionary path encourages the playful innocence of the child. Children are such fast learners because they engage all their senses with curiosity and awe. The child learns most effectively through an immersive adventure of trial and error. As adults, it's just as essential for us to nourish our childlike spark of aliveness within. With our intuitive sixth sense, we can recognize our spiritual quest in the most routine occurrences.

I continued to find profound meaning in steadfast reminders from Don Sinchi and his lineage. Instead of fantasizing about my happy places, I was instructed again and again not to avoid discomfort but to learn how to be open and at ease with all that bothered me.

Going through the many dimensions of healing simultaneously, I continued realizing the truth as a state of pure being and my fundamental essence. Emerging from old patterns and regaining new levels of vitality also involved periods of crisis.

After some time into my stay, a deep sadness came over me. This sadness felt so much greater than myself and everything that could've generated it in my brief existence. I felt immense grief for the collective suffering of all beings throughout time and space. All in all, I was engulfed in a dark cloud of despair for three months. While I was in the midst of it, however, I often felt like it would never go away.

Don Sinchi skillfully guided me to consciously allow it to run its course, no matter how fearsome it appeared. Becoming aware of the greater suffering in the world was part of Nature's wisdom—it meant that I could no longer grant myself a special place because of my own misfortunes.

The spiritual discipline of Evolutionary Science is about riding the waves of all our experiences and bringing ourselves back to wholeness by learning to abide in the openness of the heart, no matter what. Throughout this journey, I learned the power of forgiveness, which is one of the greatest gifts of an open heart. I learned to forgive others for all that they had done to me and to forgive myself for all I had done to others as well as to myself.

The inability to forgive, as Don Sinchi taught me, is a monster that drains humanity of vital life energy. Forgiveness is about learning from life experience rather than regretting it. To release all the toxicity accumulated over the years, one must simply open up to and fully feel it, without clinging to any stories, labels, or words, because true understanding takes place on the level of being.

As Don Sinchi often said, "Go beyond rejection or acceptance, beyond judgments of good or bad. It's up to you to consciously cultivate forgiveness as a continuous state that is part of your innocence and intrinsic health."

Throughout all my months in the rainforest, the higher purpose of my sickness had been steadily revealing itself. I could finally see my dis-ease as a blessing in disguise, reminding me to seek a way beyond suffering, back to the heart's wisdom. The ancestral guidance I received from the Yahua elder was about being more generous and compassionate with myself, while simultaneously standing for the truth within.

It was a great revelation for me to witness the entire universe sustained by the highest purpose of the shared heart. Seeds of fearless love had been planted within each one of us at our conception. I could see that honoring the innocence of the inner child could enable those seeds to blossom into the wisdom of compassion and truth.

The wisdom of Don Sinchi's Evolutionary Science was verified through many generations, and it completely coincided with my own intuitive insights. From those six months in the rainforest, during which my illness "magically" receded (now being in remission for 20 years), my conceptual mind's desire to "know" was replaced by the kind of profound confirmation that could only come with experience. My trust and gratitude for the living wisdom lineage of the enlightened ancestors became the basis of all the adventures that were still to come.

Tool: The Wisdom of No Escape

During the period of depression that I went through, I asked Don Sinchi how to deal with the feeling of immense suffering, which seemed to have no end. He informed me that the problem with depression, and other similar disorders of the mind and heart, is our fear of experiencing it fully, or even considering such a possibility. To dive headfirst, guided by the heart's wisdom through the dark realm of your shadows, is the wisdom of no escape. Such a daring feat requires a good, long glimpse into the radiant nature of reality beyond the conceptual mind.

The vicious cycle of mental conditioning can turn our rivers of energy into a swamp. The source of greatest joy is found in the radiance of an open heart, which is powerful beyond our perceived identities and life circumstances.

Notice whether you find yourself justifying old habits of feeling sorry for yourself or seeking excuses for staying happy. Don Sinchi taught me that the only way never to lose yourself is to avoid making a story out of your experiences, whether you consider them "good" or "bad."

Throughout your life—in every waking moment and also in your dreams (which will come with greater ease as you integrate the dreaming wave practice)—see whether you can allow all your feelings and emotions to be like the ebbs and flows of the great ocean. You can refer back to the Unlocking Your Energetic Vortexes exercise in Chapter 9 to continue to embody equanimity. The only way to release your grasp on emotional energy is *not to push away what you don't like and not to grasp what you like. If intense or difficult moments arise, don't justify your reactive emotions—instead, open yourself fully to the experience. When happiness comes, do the same thing. Only as a clear channel of Universal Love will you be able to fully heal yourself.*

REFLECTIONS

- Don Sinchi helped me access the meaning behind the big dreams that tied together so many of the major themes on my own evolutionary healing journey. As I integrated them into my understanding, I was awestruck by the way this new insight led to major transformations. *Have you had any big dreams that helped you contextualize your life's major themes in potent ways? What were they? How did they help you make sense of your healing path?*

- I learned that finding a way back to our primordial innocence is the true beginning of mapping our inner wilderness and exploring the riches that live inside us. *Do you still have any remaining fears about opening up to the childlike wisdom that lives inside you? What are the anchor memories of support you hold dear as you awaken to your innocence?*

- Change, the inevitable constant, is something few people welcome with gusto. Many of us, in the face of change, attempt to maintain a fixed identity and resist our circumstances, which only ends up hurting us and draining us of our power. The unwavering wisdom of our heart is capable of recognizing that change is nourishment, because it helps our awareness to be fresh, exponential, timeless, and eternal. *How do you generally respond to change? Can you remember the times when you braved great change with grace and were initiated into aspects of your essence that you hadn't previously known? In what ways can you commit to remaining steadfast yet flexible when change comes your way?*

- Even after the extraordinary shifts I went through in the rainforest, I still found myself having challenging experiences. I learned to accept that the healing journey is not linear, and that various layers of our human experience will come up so that we can face them and continue to recognize our true essence in the midst of them. Don Sinchi taught me that spiritual progress is not about everything being great in my life, but about how my spirit can keep shining in the face of adversity. *Can you remember times of great struggle that followed big openings on your healing journey? Instead of seeing these moments as "bad," how can you reframe them as possibilities for progress and learning on your path?*

CONCLUSION

The treasury of human potential that's been confirmed by the experience of many generations cannot be bought, stolen, or acquired by force. Without the practical approach of living wisdom, embodied by real people, it's rare to directly glimpse the transcendent human potential that's depicted in religious, philosophical, and spiritual texts. To continuously sustain such a glimpse is even harder. I was fortunate to receive that glimpse for a period that was long enough to entirely transform my life.

Ancestral pathways of experiential insight into the nature of existence from all around the world were the wellsprings that gave birth to human civilization. These embodied insights were venerated above all else within the cultural context of the ancient world. This is no longer the case.

As I learned in my journeys with Don Sinchi, ancestral wisdom was never about collecting a bag of tricks, filled with the conceptual baggage of spiritual bypassing that's so common in our world today. Genuine relatedness, self-inquiry, and discernment are some of the essential qualities that make it possible for each of us to tap into the Evolutionary Science that is humanity's birthright. Intercultural bridges, so needed now, naturally arise when we trace the original purpose of all cultures on Earth to the resilience of the noble heart in the face of adversity.

One rare advantage of globalization is easier access to wisdom traditions from around the world. If the dots are connected skillfully, the resulting evolution of a single individual's spiritual journey can be so much more effective and meaningful. When engaging a spiritual path wholeheartedly, many seemingly disparate traditions can complement one another, allowing for a more embodied insight into the nature of reality.

Unfortunately, today, due to the exploitation of natural resources, the connection with the organic intelligence of our planet is being rapidly lost within mainstream society. Drastic environmental, societal, and psychological changes are also impacting Indigenous communities. The Indigenous people have learned to adapt over millennia by mirroring their environment. When tourists come to them with a consumerist mindset, the healers reflect that back and provide the entertainment people are seeking. Nowadays, few wish to go through the arduous process of facing and transforming themselves, which causes the Indigenous traditions to become diluted. Many are now training to facilitate the Indigenous rites of Ayahuasca, which can be healing to some extent, but the original depth and potential of the ancient healing arts is being lost at an unprecedented rate.

The Indigenous elders often lack the next generation of recipients for their lineage transmission. The new generation of Indigenous people are becoming lost in an imitation of Western values, and many are ashamed to admit they are Indigenous within the general population; they even consider their own heritage to be quackery, only useful as a performance for tourists. Many elders willingly shared their life experience with me because they wholeheartedly wished for all of humanity to stay connected with the higher purpose of life, which is free of identities and comparison and allows each individual's talents to be shared fully for the benefit of the entire community. I deeply honor these glimpses of original ancestral wisdom that have been entrusted to me to share with the world.

Approaching ancestral wisdom with discernment awakens our infinite potential in the most practical and beneficial ways. It is no coincidence that ancestral guidance is emerging at this point in history, when humanity and our planet need it the most. According to many elders of the Amazon and the Andes, as well as many world traditions, these insights were destined to be revealed in today's world and applied on a massive scale as a saving grace.

Despite these inspiring possibilities, however, humanity's wisdom treasury must be approached with the utmost respect, caution, and mindfulness. Various misconceptions, superstitions, and dogmas are only some of the most common pitfalls that many encounter within the diversity of ancient traditions and healing practices. I hope this book has offered a guide as to how you can begin to skillfully integrate and utilize some of the most essential spiritual tools, especially if you wish to be part of humanity's next evolutionary leap.

Throughout my healing journey in the rainforest, I was encouraged by the elders to meet every novel concept and teaching with a grain of salt. Another essential piece of advice from the elders was to see something worth learning in everyone—even if the lesson is on how *not* to do things. To weave ancestral wisdom into the modern mindset, we must be willing to face reality beyond our comfort zone, which certainly includes interactions with difficult people and situations. This is part of the initiation into awakening our hearts to Universal Consciousness.

To effectively apply the ancestral wisdom of the Indigenous Evolutionary Science in today's world, we must recognize major differences in our worldviews. There is a gap between the intuitive, animistic cognition of the ancestors that Indigenous people still live by and the modern, rationalist frame of conceptual thinking. The living wisdom can only be shared by honoring the differences and making space for mutual learning. Without such an approach, navigating the mystical labyrinths of Indigenous mystery schools can be perilous, difficult, and confusing.

I was specifically drawn to deepen my understanding of Indigenous wisdom because I felt it held the key I'd been seeking for years. Driven by the prospect of untimely death connected to my Crohn's disease diagnosis, I wished to not only resolve my own personal suffering but also get to the root of all suffering that affects everyone indiscriminately. What initially began on a vague, intuitive level as the need for a purpose greater than myself gradually evolved into a conscious dedication to honoring the ancestral healing arts in service to all of humanity.

Immersed in the Evolutionary Science of the Amazonian healing tradition, it took me eight months to heal from the supposedly incurable disease that had initially brought me there. The resolution of that condition required prolonged periods of contact with a number of native healers, as well as drastic dietary changes and deep emotional introspection. The introspection was an essential facet of the physical purification, as releasing toxins inevitably triggered suppressed emotional content, and vice versa. The mental, emotional, and physical detox ignited in me a deep inquiry into the nature of reality as an experiential state of being that I'd never known was possible.

In light of my healing and newfound well-being, I could find no better purpose than to dedicate my life to these living wisdom traditions and apprentice with their respective lineage holders. Ever since, my motivation for walking this path has been to share the transformation, insights, and healing I experienced with those who are open to the possibility of ultimate freedom from physical, psychological, and existential suffering. These insights are at the heart of the book you have in your hands—and I hope they will propel you on your own evolutionary journey.

After years of weaving the individual threads of wisdom collected from many Amazonian elders together, I've glimpsed profound insights into the evolutionary blueprint for awakening our greatest human potential. But all those insights would not have made sense if I hadn't first learned that the spiritual path is about finding the sacredness in everything and everyone. It's not about creating "sacred cows" in the form of teachers and traditions, which defeats the entire purpose of cultivating the clarity to guide our path and dispel any illusions.

I recall a Zen teaching in which a monk tells a student that it's possible to learn something from everyone and to thus see the teacher in everyone. At the same time, we are all human, and as such, we are each sure to have our own set of limitations, ignorance, and problems dealing with the world.

The guidance of the Indigenous elders, which you've uncovered for yourself in this book, must be verified against the many trials and tribulations of life in order to genuinely awaken your human potential. To serve as a springboard for humanity to keep evolving, the Amazonian traditions I've written about here necessitate a living initiation into the mystery school of life. This can only be done through a sincere friendship with real people who've authenticated the ancient ways via their own direct and integral experience.

Do you have wise elder friends or practitioners with more experience than you in your life? The Paititi Institute hosts online and in-person retreats in the Amazon and the Andes of Peru every year, where you can undergo these initiations. I invite you to continue to explore opportunities to deepen your spiritual journey with the help of beloved community and spiritual friends who will serve to remind you of your true nature and catalyze your potential.

May your exploration of Evolutionary Science continue to bear fruit and plant seeds that flourish!

FINAL REFLECTIONS

Now that we are at the end of this book, please reflect on any transformations, subtle or overt, that you have noticed. Are you feeling a sense of reciprocity and connection between your inner and outer worlds? How has your perception of your reality changed?

Let's revisit the three pillars of this journey pointed out in the Introduction of this book:

- Understand the different unprocessed emotional energies that unconsciously determine the choices that have contributed to your everyday experiences ("getting lost in the jungle").

    Do you have a better understanding of where you get lost in the inner jungle?

    Which of your recurring patterns leads to greater anguish?

    How have your habitual patterns changed, if at all, over the course of reading this book?

- The more you become familiar with the adversities and afflictions in your life and see the degree to which they're ingrained, the more clearly you can assess what your challenges are and what's realistically required to overcome them.

    Are you beginning to use your creativity in ways that counteract the ways you get lost in the jungle? If so, how?

    Often, it takes a great deal of trial and error, and the commission of the same mistake over and over, to catch ourselves and take a different path. With the cultivation of self-kindness and acceptance, what are the new choices you are committed to making as you deepen on your own spiritual journey?

- While the first two steps prepare you to acknowledge and become aware of the task at hand, the third step allows you to uncover the spark of motivation significant enough to encourage continuous, sustained effort, which is so essential on the journey of self-realization.

Many who are on a spiritual path will have powerful realizations—from meditation, the use of plant medicines, and other sacred technologies—but stop short of transformation because they cannot maintain the stamina and motivation to continue. How is your spiritual stamina? What have you noticed about your energy to sustain the spark of innocence as a serious spiritual practice?

In the case of flagging spirits and motivation, what are the touchstones you'll rely on for strength on your journey (e.g., teachers, community, routines and practices, etc.)?

In 2010, my wife, Cynthia Robinson, and I co-founded a nonprofit organization in Peru: the Paititi Institute for the Preservation of Ecology and Indigenous Culture, which is primarily dedicated to:

- Study, restoration, and honoring the wisdom of the ancestors as a practical way to empower the Indigenous people in maintaining their heritage and ecology

- Development of intercultural bridges that demonstrate the efficacy of ancient wisdom in resolving the inner and outer causes of suffering, relevant to current critical times across our planet

Our nonprofit stewards and protects a nature reserve bordering the area of the Manu National Park, where some of the last remaining uncontacted tribes in South America live to this day. For this purpose, Paititi Institute legally owns a land title for 3,700 acres of essential watershed to the Amazon basin in the protective buffer zone of the national park.

Sustainability and the regeneration of native cultures in today's world also involves legal support to ward off mining, logging, and gold-digging activities by corrupt industries and officials. The proceeds from this book, alongside our institute's international and Peruvian-based retreats and online courses, go toward many initiatives that empower the sovereignty of Indigenous nations.

ACKNOWLEDGMENTS

My deepest gratitude ripples out to all who contributed to this book since I started writing it 17 years ago.

All my love goes to my parents and all my biological ancestors for creating the essential foundation to continue the intergenerational healing quest.

From the depth of my heart, I thank the Indigenous elders as well as my mestizo teachers for keeping the intuitive essence of enlightened ancestors alive and relevant for today's world.

I am so thankful to my dear wife and my two most amazing boys for nudging me to keep sharing about the ways of the Amazonian ancients over the years.

I wish to heartfelt thank everyone in the global community of Paititi Institute for honoring and for making a real difference in the modern world with ancestral wisdom shared in this book for so many years now.

I would like to thank The Sacred Science documentary film director Nick Polizzi for his willingness to "get real" and share about the work of the nonprofit I helped co-found with the native healers of the rainforest engaging in ancestral healing arts of illnesses today.

My deep thank you to the Hay House and Sally Mason-Swaab who has so graciously supported the publication process as well as the editor that I was assigned to Nirmala Nataraj—our synchronistic and synergistic connection made the book so much clearer and more relatable, finalizing what my elders helped me envision as a rite of passage that the reader gets to experience for themselves.

I wish to extend special thanks to all my friends who helped with beta-testing edits for two years—that process was a profound transformational experience in itself.

And last but not least, I wish to thank you, the reader for embarking on this journey to the heart of the Amazonian rainforest and rekindling your heart calling to fulfill a greater purpose in life.

ABOUT THE AUTHOR

Roman Hanis has been working closely with the Indigenous Peruvian cultures in the Amazonian rainforest and Andean mountains since 2001. During this time, he has devoted this life to learning the ancient healing ways of these cultures while seeking possibilities for creating ecological sources of sustenance for local populations and working to preserve the rainforest and its spiritual heritage of sacred medicinal plants. In 2002, Roman was fortunate enough to be cured of a terminal genetic illness, Crohn's disease. In 2004, he was pledged as a healer-curandero by the Yahua tribe and has served the international community as a medicine man ever since.

Website: **paititi-institute.org**

We hope you enjoyed this Hay House book. If you'd like to receive our online catalog featuring additional information on Hay House books and products, or if you'd like to find out more about the Hay Foundation, please contact:

Hay House LLC, P.O. Box 5100, Carlsbad, CA 92018-5100
(760) 431-7695 or (800) 654-5126
www.hayhouse.com® • www.hayfoundation.org

———

Published in Australia by:
Hay House Australia Publishing Pty Ltd
18/36 Ralph St., Alexandria NSW 2015
Phone: +61 (02) 9669 4299
www.hayhouse.com.au

Published in the United Kingdom by:
Hay House UK Ltd
1st Floor, Crawford Corner,
91–93 Baker Street, London W1U 6QQ
Phone: +44 (0)20 3927 7290
www.hayhouse.co.uk

Published in India by:
Hay House Publishers (India) Pvt Ltd
Muskaan Complex, Plot No. 3,
B-2, Vasant Kunj, New Delhi 110 070
Phone: +91 11 41761620
www.hayhouse.co.in

———

Let Your Soul Grow

Experience life-changing transformation—one video at a time—with guidance from the world's leading experts.

www.healyourlifeplus.com

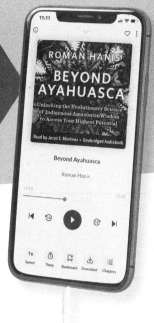

Join the Hay House E-mail Community, Your Ultimate Resource for Inspiration

Stay inspired on your journey—Hay House is here to support and empower you every step of the way!

Sign up for our **Present Moments Newsletter** to receive weekly wisdom and reflections directly from Hay House CEO Reid Tracy. Each message offers a unique perspective, grounded in Reid's decades of experience with Hay House and the publishing industry.

As a member of our e-mail community, you'll enjoy these benefits:

- **Inspiring Insights:** Discover new perspectives and expand your personal transformation with content, tips, and tools that will uplift, motivate, and inspire.

- **Exclusive Access:** Connect with world-renowned authors and experts on topics that support your journey of self-discovery and spiritual enrichment.

- **Early Updates:** Get the latest information on new and best-selling books, audiobooks, card decks, online courses, events, and more.

- **Special Offers:** Enjoy periodic announcements about discounts, limited-time offers, and giveaways.

- **Ongoing Savings:** Receive 20% off virtually all products in our online store, all day, every day, as long as you're a newsletter subscriber.

Don't miss out on this opportunity to elevate your journey with Hay House! ***Sign Up Now!***

Visit **www.hayhouse.com/newsletters** to sign up today!